ESSENTIALS
of
PHARMACY LAW

CRC PRESS
**PHARMACY
EDUCATION**
SERIES

Pharmacy: What It Is and How It Works
Peter N. Kelly

Pharmacokinetic Principles of Dosing Adjustments: Understanding the Basics
Ronald Schoenwald

Strauss's Federal Drug Laws and Examination Review, Fifth Edition
Stephen Strauss

Pharmaceutical and Clinical Calculations, Second Edition
Mansoor Khan and Indra Reddy

Inside Pharmacy: Anatomy of a Profession
Ray Gosselin, Jack Robbins, and Joseph Cupolo

*Understanding Medical Terms: A Guide for Pharmacy Practice,
Second Edition*
Mary Stanaszek, Walter Stanaszek, and Robert Holt

Pharmacokinetic Analysis: A Practical Approach
Peter Lee and Gordon Amidon

Guidebook for Patient Counseling
Harvey Rappaport, Tracey Hunter, Joseph Roy, and Kelly Straker

ESSENTIALS
of
PHARMACY LAW

DOUGLAS J. PISANO

NO LONGER THE PROPERTY
OF THE
UNIVERSITY OF R.I. LIBRARY

CRC PRESS

Boca Raton   London   New York   Washington, D.C.

Library of Congress Cataloging-in-Publication Data

Pisano, Douglas J.
    Essentials of pharmacy law / by Douglas J. Pisano.
        p. cm. — (CRC Press pharmacy education series)
    Includes bibliographical references and index.
    ISBN 1-56676-918-3 (alk. paper)
    1. Pharmacy—Law and legislation—United States. 2. Pharmacists—Legal status, laws,
etc.—United States. 3. Drugs—Law and legislation—United States. I. Title. II. Series.

KF2915.P4 P57 2002
344.73'0416—dc21   2002025927

This book contains information obtained from authentic and highly regarded sources. Reprinted material is quoted with permission, and sources are indicated. A wide variety of references are listed. Reasonable efforts have been made to publish reliable data and information, but the author and the publisher cannot assume responsibility for the validity of all materials or for the consequences of their use.

Neither this book nor any part may be reproduced or transmitted in any form or by any means, electronic or mechanical, including photocopying, microfilming, and recording, or by any information storage or retrieval system, without prior permission in writing from the publisher.

The consent of CRC Press LLC does not extend to copying for general distribution, for promotion, for creating new works, or for resale. Specific permission must be obtained in writing from CRC Press LLC for such copying.

Direct all inquiries to CRC Press LLC, 2000 N.W. Corporate Blvd., Boca Raton, Florida 33431.

Trademark Notice: Product or corporate names may be trademarks or registered trademarks, and are used only for identification and explanation, without intent to infringe.

Visit the CRC Press Web site at www.crcpress.com

© 2003 by CRC Press LLC

No claim to original U.S. Government works
International Standard Book Number 1-56676-918-3
Library of Congress Card Number 2002025927
Printed in the United States of America 2 3 4 5 6 7 8 9 0
Printed on acid-free paper

Preface

Essentials of Pharmacy Law has been written as a handy reference to be used by students at schools and colleges of pharmacy across the United States. It is designed to be of assistance to practicing pharmacists, those seeking licensure by reciprocity, and other interested healthcare professionals. The topics covered in *Essentials of Pharmacy Law* are covered in a simple and concise format. It is a compilation and commentary of selected laws and regulations pertaining to the general practice of pharmacy in the United States. It is *not* intended to take the place of an actual reading of the Laws of the United States of America, the regulations of the United States Drug Enforcement Administration, the United States Food and Drug Administration, any Board of Pharmacy, nor any department that regulates the practice of pharmacy.

About the Author

Douglas J. Pisano is an Associate Professor of Pharmacy Administration and the Dean of the newly established Massachusetts College of Pharmacy and Health Sciences, Worcester Campus. The mission of the Worcester Campus is to educate future pharmacists to be advanced level clinical practitioners with special emphasis on community practice.

In addition, he serves as the Director of the Master of Science degree program in Regulatory Affairs and Health Policy at the Boston Campus of the college. Since the Fall of 1984, he has maintained a full-time faculty appointment and is a member of the graduate faculty.

Dr. Pisano earned a Bachelor of Science degree in Pharmacy from the Massachusetts College of Pharmacy and Health Sciences, and state licensure in 1981. He earned his Master of Science degree in Public Policy/Public Affairs from the John W. McCormack Institute, University of Massachusetts at Boston in 1989, and a Doctor of Philosophy degree in Law, Policy and Society from Northeastern University in 1997.

His graduate and undergraduate teaching responsibilities include required courses in pharmacy law, FDA regulation, pharmacy management, and health policy. In 1999, Dr. Pisano was the recipient of the Trustee's Award for Teaching Excellence. In 2000, he received the Special Recognition Award for Increasing Understanding of Regulatory Affairs from the Regulatory Affairs Professionals Society.

Professor Pisano has numerous professional and peer-reviewed publications to his credit including "The Practical Guide to Pharmacy Law Series," continuing education programs, two books, and numerous chapters in areas relating to pharmacy law, drug regulation, professional malpractice, risk management, drug utilization review, health policy, and other topics in healthcare. He also has one book in development.

Professor Pisano's research interests and grants cover studies in legal/regulatory issues, cost effectiveness, professional malpractice, pharmacist/patient communications, and healthcare practice dilemmas.

A national speaker and invited lecturer, Dr. Pisano has made several hundred presentations to varied audiences of pharmacy and nonpharmacy professionals, including the Judiciary Committee of the United States House of Representatives, on the areas of pharmacy education, state and federal pharmacy, drug and device law and regulation, professional liability, pharmacy practice, health policy, and other related topics.

Contents

**Chapter 6   Pharmaceutical care: Our legal and professional
              strategic plan**

Part 2:   Case studies in pharmacy law

Chapter 7   Case studies

Part 3:   Exam review questions

Part 4:   DEA forms

part one

Introduction to pharmacy law

chapter one

The evolution of pharmacy practice

Introduction

Pharmacy, unlike chemistry or biology, is certainly not a pure science. Rather, it is a profession comprising a wide array of academic and professional disciplines that include basic sciences, business, sociology, and law. Pharmacy practice has changed as rapidly as any other profession in recent decades. In the not so distant past, a pharmacist's responsibilities were heavily concentrated in compounding and preparing a variety of medicinal dosage forms. A pharmacist would routinely prepare tablets, capsules, suppositories, elixirs, and other medicinal nostrums on the direction of the physician. However, as the pharmaceutical industry expanded, the more commonly compounded prescription products became commercially available. Neighborhood pharmacists were generally seen to augment physicians and became important providers of medical services. By the year 2000, pharmacists were increasingly more involved with therapeutic selection, drug regimen review and monitoring, and patient compliance through education and counseling.

Since ancient times, pharmacists belonged to a class of society that prepared medicines for another group who prescribed or administered them (physicians). In colonial America, the apothecary functioned as both physician and pharmacist. As drugs themselves became more complicated to make or "compound," apothecaries needed to acquire more and better skills to make them, hence, "druggists." "Compounder pharmacists" were recognized for their expertise in the formulation of the product and the physicians for their expertise relating to the patient and drug effects.[1]

After World War II, the emphasis of pharmacist practice changed from a compounder or formulator to a "technical pharmacist" whose expertise was in product distribution systems. Large pharmaceutical companies emerged with enormous technological and financial resources. They researched and developed more advanced drug products that required pharmacists to develop higher levels of professional skills and expertise. The newer products saved lives on a monumental scale, yet the chances of injury or death from the slightest medication error increased proportionately.[2]

By the 1960s, the role of extemporaneously compounding medications diminished while the need for drug therapy monitoring and patient education on drug use rose. Treating medical conditions with drug products was now called "pharmacotherapeutics," and the complexities of the therapeutic drug entities prompted patients to seek information and advice from several different practitioners. This resulted in adverse drug effects happening more often; hence, the "clinical pharmacist" was born to monitor and sometimes coordinate multiple drug therapies (polypharmacy).

During the last 20 years, the pharmacist's new role as a therapeutic advisor and overseer of drug therapy has continued to grow. The role of therapeutic advisor manifests itself primarily in the hospital setting where the opportunity to utilize medical records is presented. The drug therapy overseer role exists in the community by virtue of the patient profile that allows the pharmacist to evaluate the multiple medications that more often than not are prescribed by several different physicians. This individual is an "advocacy pharmacist." An advocacy pharmacist assumes a truly patient-oriented role to serve the patient's best interests.

Clinical pharmacy practitioners paved the way for the pharmacist's advocacy role. Because they tended to work very closely with the physician and healthcare team, they prided themselves on exceedingly high professional standards and sophisticated drug knowledge. However, the world of the clinical pharmacist is in the acute care institution and academia. Today, these same precepts have crossed into all pharmacy practice in that pharmacists who practice in the advocacy model put the patient first and discuss the benefits and detriments of medications. They encourage patients to assume responsibility for their medications based on the framework of the patient's life style, values, and environment.[3]

Meeting the challenge

In the past 20 years, the technological changes affecting the profession have been dramatic. New therapeutic entities based on biotechnology as well as diagnostic and treatment modalities have expanded. Medical specialties have also become more complex. To meet these challenges, pharmacy education has also grown. Since the opening of the Philadelphia College of Pharmacy in 1822 and the Massachusetts College of Pharmacy in Boston in 1823, 81 additional colleges of pharmacy have opened in the United States. Fewer than ten are independent, with the remainder connected to large state or private university structures. The typical pharmacy curriculum takes 6 years to complete[4] by offering the 6-year Doctor of Pharmacy degree or

Pharm.D., a terminal degree, in lieu of the Bachelor of Science offered since the 1930s.[5] In addition, many Pharm.D. holders complete hospital- or community-based residencies or research fellowships to further practice specialization in pharmacotherapeutics or clinical research.

Accreditation for pharmacy schools is awarded by the American Council on Pharmaceutical Education (ACPE), a branch of the American Association of Colleges of Pharmacy (AACP), the national association of pharmacy educational institutions. Pharmacy's primary professional association, the American Pharmaceutical Association (APhA), was founded in 1852[6] and was the first established and largest professional association of pharmacists in the United States. The APhA has more than 50,000 members including practicing pharmacists, pharmaceutical scientists, pharmacy students, pharmacy technicians, and others interested in advancing the profession. Pharmacists are licensed by state boards that administer a national exam developed by the National Association of Boards of Pharmacy.

The expanded role

Generally, a pharmacist conducts and is involved in many activities that impact and affect healthcare delivery. The principal functions of a pharmacist are preparing and dispensing of prescription medications and medical devices. Since pharmacists must be certain of the correct medication, dosage form, and directions for use prior to filling a prescription, a profile of a patient's drug therapy may be crucial to assure that the medication has appropriate instructions and is used correctly. This involvement may include the use of healthcare information. Patient counseling has also become a rapidly growing function of pharmacists because of their specialized training.

Essentially, the catalyst for these expanded functions was embodied in a very broad piece of legislation that has had great effect on the day-to-day practice of pharmacy. This legislation, passed by the United States Congress in 1990 in an outside section of the Omnibus Budget Reconciliation Act (OBRA'90), is entitled "The Medicaid Prudent Pharmaceutical Purchasing Act of 1990."[7] OBRA'90 requires pharmacists to offer counseling to Medicaid patients on all new prescriptions. The legislation establishes, codifies, and defines the criteria of proper prescription drug counseling, patient profile screening, prescription drug monitoring, and follow-up. Through some fairly sophisticated though common software, pharmacists are expected, and in Massachusetts required,[8] to monitor for potential allergies, drug interactions, drug use review, as well as inappropriate drug use or abuse. In effect, the legislation forces the pharmacist patient relationship by requiring pharmacists to interact or intervene on the behalf of the patients. At present, all state governments[9] have established their own versions of these regulations, which generally require the pharmacist to offer counseling to every patient on all new filled prescriptions.

Pharmacy's practice settings

A general snapshot of the pharmacy environment can be found in the "Survey of Pharmacy Law" which is compiled and published by the National Association of Boards of Pharmacy (NABP).[10] The United States has approximately 68,000 licensed pharmacies. Some 8000 are licensed as hospitals or institutions, 23,400 are independent pharmacies, and 13,000 are chains.*

Pharmacy, like medicine, has had to adjust to myriad sociodemographic influences. Society as a whole has become busier and more complex which has resulted in a changing emphasis in marketing pharmacy services. Accessibility, convenience, and home healthcare services are now of increased importance. These changes stem from a variety of factors such as the increase in two-income households, the growing elderly population, an increase in average life expectancy, consumer desire for convenience, and the growth of third-party insurance coverage for prescription drugs.

To adjust to these social and market influences, pharmacy has many types of practice settings. Each one is dynamic and subject to the same influences as other healthcare settings. Independent community pharmacies have long been considered by many to be among the pillars of a community; they were typically open long hours with pharmacists always available to address a variety of public health concerns. Today's independent pharmacies tend to specialize in home healthcare services, boutique compounding, durable medical equipment, or long-term care services. For example, in addition to the daily dispensing functions, a pharmacy that services a nursing home will also supply durable medical equipment, general house stock items, intravenous and enteral feeding supplies, routine medication inspections, patient profile review, staff education and in-servicing, drug use reviews, and regulation compliance. In addition, there has been an initiative to develop other professional cognitive services concerning cholesterol, hypertension, diabetes, occult fecal blood, and hearing loss, in all community practice settings.

Chain pharmacies are also quite prevalent and generally outnumber independent pharmacies by a ratio of 3:1. Chain pharmacies usually have ten or more retail outlets that operate under a single corporate banner. Chain pharmacies typically have greater product selection due to larger facilities and buying power, a perception of lower price, and large health and beauty aid departments along with high-volume prescription services. Supermarket pharmacies are considered chain pharmacies by having successfully included prescription departments within supermarket or grocery-type stores. The main offering of supermarket/combination type pharmacy settings is the convenience of one-stop shopping for the majority of a consumer's needs.

---

* Five states include the number of chain pharmacists in the community-independent pharmacist figure. Also, information is available for only 45 states.

Mail service pharmacies are also becoming quite prevalent. Theirs is primarily a dispensing/supervisory role. In most cases, there is a contract with health insurers, national associations, and third-party payers to provide prescription and formulary services. These pharmacies potentially lower out-of-pocket expense and offer the convenience of prescriptions delivered by mail. Mail service pharmacies are considered very high-volume prescription operations (>3000 prescriptions filled per day) and pharmacists generally participate more routinely in checking prescriptions filled by technicians, rather than actually filling the prescriptions themselves, as well as making calls to physicians and answering patient questions via telephone.

Clinical and institutional pharmacy has also been evolving during the past several years. When the term "clinical pharmacist" was first used only a handful of select pharmacists fit the role. These pharmacists were initially found in large teaching hospitals associated with medical schools and they provided specialty pharmacotherapeutic services such as pharmacokinetics, infectious disease, or cardiology to name a few. Meanwhile, the typical institutional pharmacist spent time in the basement of the central pharmacy taking and filling drug orders that were sent down from the medical floors.

Eventually, pharmacy was moved from a centralized location to various places throughout the hospital. The institutional/staff pharmacists then began filling orders directly and interacting with the physicians and clinical pharmacists to help provide some pharmaceutical care. This model has continued to evolve and has spread to some of the smaller community hospitals with the institutional pharmacist gaining more of a clinical role. The pharmacist is thus seen as more than a dispenser of medication; he or she is also recognized by the healthcare system as an information resource for pharmacotherapeutic knowledge.

The widespread acceptance of the pharmacist as a purveyor of knowledge as well as of medications has led to some standardization for the provision of pharmaceutical care. The American Society of Health-System Pharmacists (ASHP) is one organization that has established a set of guidelines. These guidelines provide a systematic approach for pharmacists to use in the implementation and provision of pharmaceutical care.

The initial step in pharmaceutical care is the collection and organization of pertinent patient-specific information to develop a database to prevent, detect, and resolve a patient's medication problems. The next step is to take these data and determine the presence of medication-therapy problem(s) and assess the relative importance of each. Once this has been done, the pharmacist needs to summarize the patient's healthcare needs in relation to desired outcomes and other health professionals' assessments, goals, and therapy plans. This information is then used to design a specific pharmaco therapeutic goal to be utilized to achieve specific medication-related outcomes and improve the patient's quality of life. Once the pharmacist has implemented and established these initial guidelines, then he or she is ready to begin the next phase of pharmaceutical care.

The pharmacist, in concert with all those involved with the patient's care, will then design a pharmacotherapeutic regimen for the patient. The regimen is designed for optimal medication use within the health system's and the patient's capabilities and financial resources. After designing the plan a monitoring program for the pharmacotherapeutic regimen is developed to ensure the safety and efficacy of the regimen. This is also done in conjunction with all those involved in the patient's care.

The final steps of the process include the initiation and monitoring of the pharmacotherapeutic regimen. The pharmacist implements and monitors the success of the regimen in conjunction with the other healthcare providers. The last step is to monitor the patient's outcome and then redesign the pharmacotherapeutic regimen and plan as needed.

These standard guidelines allow the pharmacist to practice pharmaceutical care in a number of different practice settings. This expanded role is supported by the presence of pharmacists practicing pharmaceutical care in the acute care hospitals, ambulatory care and family practice clinics, long-term care facilities, and home care programs.

However, the pharmacist of the 21st century cannot practice pharmaceutical care without an intimate knowledge of medication, pharmacy practice, and the laws and regulations that govern them. Therefore, the purpose of this book is not to teach the practice of pharmacy. Rather, it is designed to assist pharmacists, pharmacy interns, and pharmacy technicians in the practical aspects of their daily professional activities by serving as a handy reference guide to answer fundamental questions of pharmacy practice and the law.

Bibliography

1. Smith, M. and Knapp, D., Pharmacy settings and types of practice, *Pharmacy, Drugs and Medical Care*, 4th ed., Lippincott, Williams & Wilkins, Philadelphia, 1987, p. 123.
2. Sonnendecker, G., *Evolution of Pharmacy*, Remington's Pharmaceutical Sciences, 5th ed., Mack Publishing, Easton, PA, p. 8.
3. Brushwood, D., The pharmacist's duty to warn: Toward a knowledge-based model of professional responsibility, *Drake Law Review*, 40, 182, 1991.
4. Fincham, J.E. and Wertheimer, A.I., *Pharmacy and the U.S. Health Care System*, Pharmaceutical Products Press, Binghamton, NY, 1991.
5. Buerki, R. and Vottaro, L., *Ethical Responsibility and Pharmacy Practice*, American Institute of the History of Pharmacy, Madison, WI, 1994, p. 2.
6. Buerki, R. and Vottaro, L., *Ethical Responsibility and Pharmacy Practice*, American Institute of the History of Pharmacy, Madison, WI, 1994, p. 146.
7. Omnibus Budget Reconciliation Act of 1990, PL. 101-508.
8. MGL. 112, Ch. 94c, Sec. 21a Patient Counseling.
9. *1999–2000 Survey of Pharmacy Law*, National Association of Boards of Pharmacy, Park Ridge, IL, p. 56.
10. *1999–2000 Survey of Pharmacy Law*, National Association of Boards of Pharmacy, Park Ridge, IL.

chapter two

U.S. drug regulation

Overview

Regulations and laws are central social constructs that provide guidance for all societies around the globe. Governments create laws in a number of ways with various intents for myriad purposes. In the United States, laws are created by Congress, a body of officials elected by the citizenry, who are charged with the governance of the country by representing the common public good. The Congress proposes and passes laws that are relatively general in nature and are intended to address some particular issue in a fashion that can be consistently applied by all who are affected by them. Once passed, laws are remanded to the appropriate government or administrative agency that then decides how these laws are to be applied. These applications of law are called regulations. Regulations serve as the practical foundation from which citizens adhere to the law as it was originally intended.

In the United States, all food, drugs, cosmetics, and medical devices for both humans and animals are regulated under the authority of the Food and Drug Administration (FDA). FDA and all of its regulations were created by the government in response to the pressing need to address the safety of the public with respect to its foods and medicinals. The purpose of this chapter is to describe and explain the nature and extent of these regulations as they apply to drugs in the United States. An historical perspective is offered as a basis for regulatory context. In addition, this chapter discusses FDA regulatory oversight and that of other agencies, the drug approval and development process, the mechanisms used to regulate manufacturing and marketing, as well as various violation and enforcement schema.

Brief history of drug laws and regulations

Prior to 1902, the U.S. government took a hands-off approach to the regulation of drugs. Many of the drugs available were so-called "patent medicines," so named because each had a more or less descriptive or patent name. No laws, regulations, or standards existed to any noticeable extend even though the United States Pharmacopeia (USP) became a reality in 1820 as the first official compendium of the United States. The USP set standards for strength and purity that could be used by physicians and pharmacists who needed centralized guidelines to extract, compound, and otherwise utilize the drug components that existed at the time.[1]

However, in 1848, the first American drug law, the Drug Importation Act, was enacted when American troops serving in Mexico became seriously ill from adulterated quinine, an anti-malarial drug, was discovered. This law required laboratory inspection, detention, and even destruction of drugs that did not meet acceptable standards. Later, in 1902, the Virus, Serum and Toxins Act (Biologics Control Act) was passed in response to tetanus-infected diphtheria antitoxin which was manufactured by a small laboratory in St. Louis, Missouri. Ten school children died as a result of the tainted serum. No national standards were as yet in place for purity or potency. The Act authorized the Public Health Service to license and regulate the interstate sale of serum, vaccines, and related biologic products used to prevent or treat disease.

This Act also spurred Dr. Harvey W. Wiley, Chief Chemist for the Bureau of Chemistry, a branch of the United States Department of Agriculture (USDA) and the forerunner for today's United States Food and Drug Administration (FDA), to investigate the country's foods and drugs. He established the Hygienic Table, a group of young men who volunteered to serve as human guinea pigs and allowed Dr. Wiley to feed them a controlled diet laced with a variety of preservatives and artificial colors. More popularly known as the "Poison Squad," they helped Dr. Wiley gather enough data to prove that many of America's foods and drugs were adulterated, that a product's strength or purity was suspect or misbranded, or had inadequate or inaccurate labeling. Dr. Wiley's efforts, along with publication of Upton Sinclair's *The Jungle* (a book revealing the putrid conditions in America's meat industry), were rewarded when Congress passed America's first food and drug law in 1906, the Pure Food and Drug Act (USPFDA) (also known as the Wiley Act). The Wiley Act prohibited interstate commerce of misbranded foods or drugs based on their labeling. It did not affect unsafe drugs because its legal authority only came to bear when a product's ingredients were falsely labeled. Even intentionally false therapeutic claims were not prohibited.

This began to change in 1911 with the enactment of the Sherley Amendment that was intended to prohibit the labeling of medications with false therapeutic claims to defraud the purchaser. These amendments, however, required the government to find proof of intentional labeling fraud. Later, in 1937, a seminal event occurred that changed the entire regulatory picture. Sulfa became the miracle drug of the time and was used to treat many life-threatening infections. It tasted bad and was hard to swallow, which led entrepreneurs to seek a palatable solution. S.E. Massingill Co. of Bristol, Tennessee developed what it thought was a palatable, raspberry-flavored liquid product. However, it used diethylene glycol to solubilize the sulfa. Six gallons of this dangerous mixture, Elixir of Sulfanilamide, killed some 107 people, mostly children.

The result was the passage of one of the most comprehensive statutes in the history of American health law. The Federal Food, Drug and Cosmetic Act of 1938 (FDCA) repealed the Sherley Amendments and required that all new drugs be tested by their manufacturers for safety who would then submit those tests to the government for marketing approval via a New Drug Application. The FDCA also mandated that drugs be labeled with adequate directions if they were shown to have had harmful effects. In addition, the FDCA authorized FDA to conduct unannounced inspections of drug manufacturing facilities. Though amended many times since 1938, the FDCA is still the broad foundation for FDA statutory authority as it exists today.

However, a new crisis loomed. Throughout the late 1950s, European and Canadian physicians began to encounter a number of infants born with a curious birth defect called "phocomeglia," a defect that resulted in limbs which resembled flippers similar to those found on seals. These birth defects were traced to mothers who had been prescribed the drug thalidomide in an effort to relieve morning sickness while pregnant. The manufacturer of this drug applied for U.S. marketing approval as a sleep aid. However, due to the efforts of Dr. Frances O. Kelsey, the FDA chief medical officer at the time, the case was made that the drug was not safe and therefore not for release the U.S. marketplace.

Dr. Kelsey's efforts and the decisive work by the U.S. Congress resulted in yet another necessary amendment to the FDCA in 1962, the Kefauver-Harris Act. This Act essentially closed many of the loopholes regarding drug safety in American law. These Drug Efficacy Amendments required drug manufacturers to prove the safety and efficacy of their drug products, register with FDA and be inspected at least every 2 years, have their prescription drug advertising approved by FDA (this authority being transferred from the Federal Trade Commission), provide and obtain documented informed consent from research subjects prior to human trials, and increase controls over manufacturing and testing to determine drug effectiveness.

In an effort to address the new provisions of the Act, the FDA contracted the National Academy of Sciences along with the National Research Council to examine some 3400 drug products approved between 1938 and 1962 based on safety alone. Called the Drug Efficacy Study Implementation Review of 1966 (DESI), it charged these organizations to make a determination as to whether post-1938 drug products were "Effective" for the indications claimed in their labeling, or "Probably Effective," "Possibly Effective," or "Ineffective." Those products not deemed "Effective" were removed from the marketplace, reformulated, or sold with a clear warning to prescribers that the product was not deemed effective.

Later, in 1972, FDA began to examine over-the-counter (OTC) drug products. Phase II of the Drug Efficacy Amendments required FDA to determine the efficacy of OTC drug products. This project was much larger in scope than the analysis of prescription drugs. In the America of the 1970s, consumers could choose from more than 300,000 OTC drug products. FDA soon realized that it did not have the resources to evaluate each and every one. Hence, FDA created advisory panels of scientists, medical professionals, and consumers who were charged with evaluating the active ingredients used in OTC products within 80 defined therapeutic categories. After examining both the scientific and medical literature of the day, the advisory panels made decisions regarding active ingredients and their labeling. The result was a monograph that described, in detail, acceptable active ingredients and labeling for products within a therapeutic class. Products that complied with monograph guidelines were deemed Category I: Safe and effective, not misbranded. However, products not in compliance with monograph guidelines were deemed Category II: Not safe and effective or misbranded. Category II products were removed from the marketplace or reformulated. Products for which data were insufficient for classification were deemed Category III and were allowed to continue on the market until substantive data could be established or until they were reformulated and in compliance with the monograph. The OTC Drug Review took approximately 20 years to complete.

Though numerous other federal laws and regulations were passed throughout the 1970s, many were based on regulating the professional practice of medical professionals or for the direct protection of consumers. For example, the Federal Controlled Substances Act (CSA), part of the Comprehensive Drug Abuse and Prevention Act of 1970, placed drugs with a relatively high potential for abuse into five federal schedules along with a closed record-keeping system designed to track federally controlled substances via a definitive paper trail as they were ordered, prescribed, dispensed, and utilized throughout the healthcare system.

Significant regulatory change also occurred in the 1980s. Biotechnology was developing on a grand scale and the pharmaceutical industry was on its cutting edge. Many of the medicinal compounds discovered were very expensive and had limited use in the general U.S. population. However, these compounds could prove life saving to demographically small patient populations who suffered from diseases and conditions that were considered rare. In an effort to encourage these biotechnical pharmaceutical companies to continue to develop these and other products, Congress passed the Orphan Drug Act in 1983. The Act continues to allow manufacturers to gain incentives for research, development, and marketing of drug products used to treat rare diseases or conditions which would otherwise be unprofitable via a system of breaks and deductions in manufacturers' corporate taxes. Though the success of the Orphan Drug Act provided great medical benefit for a few, a scandal loomed in other parts of the pharmaceutical industry.

The generic pharmaceutical industry experienced steady growth as many of the exclusive patents enjoyed by major pharmaceutical companies for brand-named products were beginning to expire. Generic versions of these now freely copied products were appearing much more frequently in the marketplace. However, these generic copies were required to undergo the same rigorous testing that brand-name, pioneer, or innovator products did. This led to a very public scandal concerning a few unscrupulous generic pharmaceutical companies that took shortcuts in reporting data, submitted fraudulent samples, and offered bribes to FDA officials to gain easy and rapid market approval of their products. As a result, Congress passed the Price Competition and Patent Restoration Act of 1984. This Act, also called the Waxman-Hatch Act after its sponsors, was designed to level the playing field in the prescription drug industry with regard to pioneer/innovator/brand-name prescription drug products and their generic copies. The Act was composed of two distinct parts or "Titles." Title I was for the benefit of the generic pharmaceutical industry. It extended the scope of the Abbreviated New Drug Application to cover generic versions of post-1962-approved drug products. It required that generic versions of pioneer or innovator drugs have the same relevant aspects with regard to bioequivalence (rate and extent of absorption of the active drug in the human body) and pharmaceutical equivalence (same dosage form as the pioneer drug to which it is compared). Though somewhat simplified, the Waxman-Hatch Act permitted easier market access to generic copies of pioneer drugs provided they were not significantly different from the pioneer drug in their absorption, action, and dosage form. In addition, Title II of the Act was designed to aid and encourage research-based or innovator pharmaceutical companies to continue their search for new and useful medicinal compounds by extending the patent life of pioneer drug products while in the FDA review period.

However, the patent extension benefit has become somewhat moot due to an overall reduction in FDA review time as a result of prescription drug user fees. In 1992, Congress passed the Prescription Drug User Fee Act (PDUFA). The Act was intended to help FDA generate additional funds to upgrade and modernize its operations and to accelerate drug approval. It authorized FDA to charge pharmaceutical manufacturers a user fee to accelerate drug review. As a result of the PDUFA legislation, FDA has been able to reduce approval time of new pharmaceutical products from greater than 30 months to approximately 13 to 15 months today. However, the Act had a "sunset" provision that limited FDA authority to charge user fees until the year 1997.

After reviewing the successes of the PDUFA legislation, Congress extended the user fee provisions during passage of the FDA Modernization Act (FDAMA) of 1997. FDMA reauthorized the fees until September 30, 2002, when they will be revisited in an effort to further reduce prescription drug approval time. However, the Act not only extended user fee provisions, it gave FDA the authority to conduct "fast track" product reviews to speed lifesaving drug therapies to market, it permitted an additional 6-month patent exclusivity for pediatric prescription drug products, and it required the National Institutes of Health to build a publicly accessible database on clinical studies of investigational drugs or life-threatening diseases.

American drug law has come quite far since the early 1900s. Today, FDA continues to work with Congress and the pharmaceutical industry to regulate and evaluate new and existing drug, biologic, and device products. The overriding regulatory challenge that FDA faces will be to keep current, through regulation and policy, with future technological advances by science and industry.

Regulatory oversight of pharmaceuticals

The primary responsibility for the regulation and oversight of pharmaceuticals and the pharmaceutical industry lies with U.S. Food and Drug Administration (FDA). FDA was created in 1931 and is one of several branches within the U.S. Department of Health and Human Services (HHS). FDA counterparts within HHS include agencies such as the Centers for Disease Control and Prevention (CDC), the National Institutes of Health (NIH), and the Healthcare Financing Administration (HCFA).

FDA is organized into a number of offices and centers headed by a commissioner who is appointed by the President with the consent of the Senate. It is a scientifically based law enforcement agency whose mission is to safeguard the public health and to ensure honesty and fairness among health-regulated industries, i.e., pharmaceutical, device, biologic, and the consumer companies.[2] It licenses and inspects manufacturing facilities, tests products, evaluates claims and prescription drug advertising, monitors research, and creates regulations, guidelines, standards, and policies. It does all of this through its Office of Operations which contains component offices and centers such as the Center for Drug Evaluation and Research (CDER), Center for Biologics Evaluation and Research (CBER), Center for Devices and Radiological Health (CDRH), Center for Food Safety and Applied Nutrition (CFSAN), the Center for Veterinary Medicine (CVM), Office of Orphan Products Development, Office of Biotechnology, Office of Regulatory Affairs, and the National Center for Toxicological Research. Each of these entities has a defined role, though sometimes their authorities overlap. For example, if a pharmaceutical company submits a drug that is contained and delivered to a patient during therapy by a device not comparable to any other, CDER and CDRH may need to coordinate that product's approval. Though most prescription drugs are evaluated by CDER, any other center or office may become involved with its review. One of the most significant resources to industry and consumers is the FDA website www.fda.gov. Easily accessible and navigable, each center and office has its own HTML within the site.

FDA is not the only agency within the U.S. government with a stake in pharmaceutical issues. The Federal Trade Commission (FTC) has authority over business practices in general such as deceptive and anti-competitive practices, i.e., false advertising. In addition, FTC regulates the advertising of OTC drugs, medical devices, and cosmetics. To a lesser degree, the Consumer Product Safety Commission (CPSC) regulates hazardous substances and the containers of poisons and other harmful agents; the Environmental

Protection Agency (EPA) regulates pesticides used in agriculture and FDA-regulated food products; the Occupational Safety and Health Administration (OSHA) regulates the working environment of employees who may use FDA-regulated commodities, i.e., syringes, chemotherapy, chemical reagents; the Healthcare Financing Administration (HCFA) regulates the federal Medicaid and Medicare programs; and the Drug Enforcement Administration (DEA) enforces the Federal Controlled Substances Act and is charged with controlling and monitoring the flow of licit and illicit controlled substances. There are also various state and local drug control agencies that establish their own regulations and procedures for manufacturing, research, and development of pharmaceuticals.

New drug approval and development

Prior to any discussion of how pharmaceuticals make their way through FDA for market approval, one needs to have an understanding of what constitutes a drug. A "drug" is a substance that exerts an action on the structure or function of the body by chemical action or metabolism and is intended for use in the diagnosis, cure, mitigation, treatment, or prevention of disease.[3] The concept of "new drug" stems from the Kefauver-Harris Amendments to the FDCA. A new drug is defined as one that is not generally recognized as safe and effective for the indications proposed. However, this definition has much greater reach than simply a new chemical entity. The term "new drug" also refers to a drug product already in existence though never approved by FDA for marketing in the United States; new therapeutic indications; a new dosage form; a new route of administration; a new dosing schedule; or any significant clinical differences other than those approved.[4] Therefore, any chemical substance intended for use in humans or animals for medicinal purposes, or any existing chemical substance that has some significant change associated with it, is considered not safe or effective and a new drug until proper testing and FDA approval occur.

FDA approval can be a fairly lengthy and expensive process. For a pharmaceutical manufacturer to place a product on the market for human use, a multiphase procedure must be followed. The mission of FDA is to protect the public and it takes that charge very seriously. Hence, all drug products must at least follow the stepwise process.

Preclinical investigation

Human testing of new drugs cannot begin until there is solid evidence that the drug product can be used with reasonable safety in humans. This phase is called "Preclinical Investigation." The basic goal of preclinical investigation is to assess potential therapeutic effects of the substance on living organisms and to gather sufficient data to determine reasonable safety of the substance in humans through laboratory experimentation and animal investigation.[5] FDA requires no prior approval for investigators or pharmaceutical industry sponsors to begin a preclinical investigation on a potential drug substance. Investigators and sponsors are, however, required to follow Good Laboratory Practice (GLP) regulations.[6] GLPs govern laboratory facilities, personnel, equipment, and operations. Compliance with GLPs requires procedures for documentation of training, study schedules, processes, and status reports which are submitted to facility management and included in the final study report to FDA. A preclinical investigation usually takes 1 to 3 years to complete. If at that time enough data are gathered to reach the goal of potential therapeutic effect and reasonable safety, the product sponsor must formally notify FDA of its wishes to test the potential new drug on humans.

Investigational New Drug Application (INDA)

Unlike the preclinical investigation stage, the INDA phase has much more direct FDA activity throughout the process. Because a preclinical investigation is designed to gather significant evidence of a compound's reasonable safety and efficacy in live organisms, the INDA is the clinical phase where all activity is used to gather significant evidence of reasonable safety and efficacy data about the potential drug compound in humans. Clinical trials in humans are carefully scrutinized and regulated by FDA to protect the health and safety of human test subjects and to ensure the integrity and usefulness of the clinical study data.[7] Numerous meetings between both the agency and sponsor will occur during this time. As a result, the clinical investigation phase may take as long as 12 years to complete. Only one in five compounds tested may actually demonstrate clinical effectiveness and safety and reach the U.S. marketplace.

The sponsor will submit the INDA to FDA. The INDA must contain information on the compound itself and information about the study. All INDAs must have the same basic components: a detailed cover sheet, a table of contents, an introductory statement and basic investigative plan, an investigators brochure, comprehensive investigation protocols, the compound's actual or proposed chemistry, manufacturing and controls, any pharmacology and toxicology information, any previous human experience with the compound, and any other pertinent information FDA deems necessary. After submission, the sponsor company must wait 30 days to commence clinical trials. If FDA does not object within that period, the trials may begin.

Prior to the actual commencement of the clinical investigations, however, a few ground rules must be established. For example, a clinical study protocol must be developed, proposed by the sponsor, and reviewed by an Institutional Review Board (IRB). An IRB is required by regulation[8] and is a committee of medical and ethical experts designated by an institution such as a university medical center in which the clinical trial will take place. The charge of the IRB is to oversee the research to ensure that the rights of human test subjects are protected and that rigorous medical and scientific standards are maintained.[7] An IRB must approve the proposed clinical study and monitor the research as it progresses. It must develop written procedures of its own regarding its study review process and its reporting of any changes to the ongoing study as they occur. In addition, an IRB must also review and approve documents for informed consent prior to commencement of the proposed clinical study. Regulations require that potential participants be informed adequately about the risks, benefits, and treatment alternatives before participating in experimental research.[9] An IRB's membership must be sufficiently diverse in order to review the study in terms of the specific research issue, community and legal standards, and professional conduct and practice norms. All of its activities must be well documented and open to FDA inspection at any time.

Once the IRB is satisfied that the proposed trial is ethical and proper, it can begin. The clinical trial has three steps or phases. Each has a purpose, requires numerous patients, and can take more than 1 year to complete.

Phase I

A Phase I study is relatively small, fewer than 100 subjects, and brief (1 year or less). Its purpose is to determine toxicology, metabolism, pharmacologic actions, and if possible any early evidence of effectiveness. The results of the Phase I study are used to develop the next step.

Phase II

Phase II studies are the first controlled clinical studies using several hundred subjects who are afflicted with the disease or condition being studied. The purpose of Phase II is to determine the compound's possible effectiveness against the targeted disease or condition and its safety in humans. Phase II may be divided into two subparts: Phase IIa which is a pilot study used to determine initial efficacy and Phase IIb which uses controlled studies on several hundred patients. At the end of Phase II studies, the sponsor and FDA will usually confer about the data and plans for Phase III.

Phase III

Phase III studies are considered pivotal trials which are designed to collect all of the necessary data to meet the safety and efficacy standards FDA requires to approve the compound for the U.S. marketplace. Phase III studies are usually very large, consisting of several thousand patients in numerous study centers with a large number of investigators who conduct long-term trials over several months or years. Also, Phase III studies establish final formulation, marketing claims and product stability, and packaging and storage conditions. On completion of Phase III, all clinical studies are complete, all safety and efficacy data have been analyzed, and the sponsor is ready to submit the compound to FDA for market approval. This process begins with submission of a New Drug Application (NDA).

New Drug Application (NDA)

An NDA is a regulatory mechanism that is designed to give FDA sufficient information to make a meaningful evaluation of a new drug.[10] All NDAs must contain the following information: preclinical laboratory and animal data; human pharmacokinetic and bioavailability data; clinical data; methods of manufacturing, processing, and packaging; a description of the drug product and substance; a list of relevant patents for the drug, its manufacture, or claims; and any proposed labeling. In addition, an NDA must provide a summary of the application's contents and a presentation of the risks and benefits of the new drug.[11] Traditionally, NDAs consisted of hundreds of volumes of information, in triplicate, all cross-referenced. Since 1999, FDA has issued final guidance documents that allow sponsors to submit NDAs electronically in a standardized format. These electronic submissions facilitate ease of review and possible approval.[12]

The NDA must be submitted complete, in the proper form and with all critical data. If accepted, FDA will then determine the application's completeness. If complete, the agency considers the application filed and will begin the review process within 60 days.[13] The purpose of an NDA from the FDA perspective is to ensure that the new drug meets the criteria to be safe and effective. Safety and effectiveness are determined through Phase III pivotal studies based on substantial evidence gained from a well-controlled clinical study. Since FDA realizes there are no absolutely safe drugs, FDA looks to the new drug's efficacy as a measure of its safety. It weighs the risks vs. benefits of approving the drug for use in the U.S. market.

Also, the NDA must be very clear about the manufacture and marketing of the proposed drug product. The application must define and describe manufacturing processes, validate Current Good Manufacturing Practices (CGMPs), provide evidence of quality, purity, strength, identity, and bioavailability (a pre-inspection of the manufacturing facility will be conducted by FDA). Finally, FDA will review all product packaging and labeling for content and clarity. Statements on a product's package label, package insert, media advertising, and professional literature must be reviewed. Of note, "labeling" refers to all of the above and not just the label on the product container.

FDA is required to review an application within 180 days of filing. At the end of that time, the agency is required to respond with an action letter. There are three kinds of action letters. An "Approval Letter" signifies that all substantive requirements for approval are met and that the sponsor company can begin marketing the drug as of the date on the letter. An "Approvable Letter" signifies that the application substantially complies with the requirements but has some minor deficiencies that must be addressed before an approval letter is sent. Generally, these deficiencies are minor in nature and the product's sponsor must respond within 10 days of receipt. At this point, the sponsor may amend the application and address the agency's concerns, request a hearing with the agency, or withdraw the application entirely.

A "Non-Approvable Letter" signifies that FDA has major concerns with the application and will not approve the proposed drug product as submitted for marketing. The remedies available for a sponsor to take for this type of action letter are similar to those in the approvable letter.

PDUFA/FDAMA effects

NDA review has been significantly affected by both PDUFA and FDAMA legislation. The Prescription Drug User Fee Act (PDUFA) allows FDA to collect fees from sponsor companies who submit applications for review. The fees are used to update facilities and hire and train reviewers. The fees only apply to NDA drug submissions, biologic drug submissions, and any supplement thereto. The fees do not apply to generic drugs or medical devices. The results of the PDUFA legislation were significant: approval rates have increased from approximately 50% to near 80% and the review times have decreased to under 15 months for most applications.[14]

Later, in 1997, the FDA Modernization Act (FDAMA) reauthorized PDUFA until the year 2002. It waives the user fee to small companies who have fewer than 500 employees and are submitting their first applications. It allows payment of the fee in stages and permits some percentage of refund if the application is refused. Also, it exempts applications for drugs used in rare conditions (orphan drugs), supplemental applications for pediatric indications, and applications for biologicals used as precursors for other biologics manufacture. In addition, FDMA permits fast track approval of compounds that demonstrate significant benefit to critically ill patients such as those who suffer from AIDS.[15]

Biologics

Biologics are defined as substances derived from or made with the aid of living organisms including vaccines, antitoxins, serums, blood, blood products, therapeutic protein drugs derived from natural sources (i.e., anti-thrombin III), or biotechnology (i.e., recombinantly derived proteins), and gene or somatic cell therapies.[16] As with the more traditionally derived drug products, biologics follow virtually the same regulatory and clinical testing schema with regard to safety and efficacy. A Biologics License Application (BLA) is used rather than an NDA, though the official FDA form is designated the 356h and is one and the same. The sponsor merely indicates in a check box if the application is for a drug or a biologic. Compounds characterized as biologics are reviewed by CBER.[17]

Orphan drugs

Orphan drugs are approved by using many of the same processes as any other application. However, there are several significant differences. An orphan drug as defined under the Orphan Drug Act of 1993 as a drug used to treat a rare disease that would not normally be of interest to commercial manufacturers in the ordinary course of business. A "rare disease" is defined in the law as any disease that affects fewer than 200,000 persons in the United States or one in which a manufacturer has no reasonable expectation of recovering the cost of its development and availability in the United States. The Act creates a series of financial incentives of which manufacturers can take advantage. For example, the Act permits grant assistance for clinical research, tax credits for research and development, and 7-year market exclusivity to the first applicant who obtains market approval for a drug designated as an orphan. This means that if a sponsor gains approval for an orphan drug, FDA will not approve any application by any other sponsor for the same drug for the same disease or condition for 7 years from the date of the first applicant's approval provided certain conditions are met, such as an assurance of sufficient availability of drug to those in need or a revocation of the drug's orphan status.[18,19]

Abbreviated New Drug Applications (ANDA)

Abbreviated New Drug Applications (ANDAs) are used when a patent has expired for a product on the U.S. market and a company wishes to market a copy. In the United States, a drug patent is for 20 years. After that time, a manufacturer is able to submit an abbreviated application for that product provided it certifies that the product patent in question has already expired, is invalid, or will not be infringed.

The generic copy must meet with certain other criteria as well. The drug's active ingredient must already be approved for the conditions of use proposed in the ANDA, and nothing must have changed to call into question the basis for approval of the original drug's NDA.[20] Sponsors of ANDAs are required to prove that their version meets the standards of bioequivalence and pharmaceutical equivalence. FDA publishes a list of all approved drugs titled the "Approved Drug Products with Therapeutic Equivalence Evaluations." It is also called the "Orange Book" because of its orange-colored cover. It lists marketed drug products that are considered by FDA to be safe and effective and provides information on therapeutic equivalence evaluations for approved multisource prescription drug products[21] monthly. The Orange Book rates drugs based on their therapeutic equivalence. For a product to be considered therapeutically equivalent, it must be both pharmaceutically equivalent (i.e., the same dose, dosage form, strength, etc.) and bioequivalent (i.e., rate and extent of its absorption are not significantly different from the absorption rate and extent of the drug with which it is to be interchanged).

Realizing that there may be some degree of variability in patients, FDA allows pharmaceuticals to be considered bioequivalent through either of two methods. The first method studies the rate and extent of absorption of a test drug that may or may not be a generic variation, and a reference or brand-name drug under similar experimental conditions in similar dosing schedules where the test results do not show significant differences. The second approach uses the same method but the results determine that there is a difference in the test drug's rate and extent of absorption, except the difference is considered to be medically insignificant for the proper clinical outcome of that drug.

> Bioequivalence of different formulations of the same drug substance involves equivalence with respect to the rate and extent of drug absorption. Two formulations whose rate and extent of absorption differ by 20% or less are generally considered bioequivalent. The use of the 20% rule is based on a medical decision that, for most drugs, a 20% difference in the concentration of the active ingredient in blood will not be clinically significant.[22]

The FDA Orange Book uses a two-letter coding system that is helpful in determining which drug products are considered therapeutically equivalent. The first letter, either an "A" or a "B," indicates a drug product's therapeutic equivalence rating. The second letter describes dose forms and can be any one of a number of different letters.

The A codes are described in the Orange Book as follows:

> Drug products that FDA considers to be therapeutically equivalent to other pharmaceutically equivalent products, i.e., drug products for which:
>
> 1. There are no known or suspected bioequivalence problems. These are designated AA, AN, AO, AP or AT, depending on the dose form; or
>
> 2. Actual or potential bioequivalence problems have been resolved with adequate *in vivo* and/or *in vitro* evidence supporting bioequivalence. These are designated AB.[24]

The B codes are a much less desirable rating when compared to an A rating. Products rated B may still be commercially marketed; however, they may not be considered therapeutically equivalent. The Orange Book describes B codes as follows:

> Drug products that FDA at this time does not consider to be therapeutically equivalent to other pharmaceutically equivalent products, i.e., drug products for which actual or potential bioequivalence problems have not been resolved by adequate evidence of bioequivalence. Often the problem is with specific dosage forms rather

than with the active ingredients. These are designated
BC, BD, BE, BN, BP, BR, BS, BT, or BX.[24]

FDA has adopted an additional subcategory of B codes. The designation B* is assigned to former A-rated drugs "if FDA receives new information that raises a significant question regarding therapeutic equivalence."[25] Not all drugs are listed in the Orange Book. Drugs obtainable only from a single manufacturing source, DESI-drugs, or drugs manufactured prior to 1938 are not included. Those that do appear are listed by generic name.

Phase IV and post-marketing surveillance

Pharmaceutical companies that successfully gain marketing approval for their products are *not* exempt from further regulatory requirements. Many products are approved for market on the basis of continued submission of clinical research data to FDA. These data may be required to further validate efficacy or safety, detect new uses or abuses for the product, or to determine the effectiveness of labeled indications under conditions of widespread usage.[26] FDA may also require a Phase IV study for drugs approved under the FDAMA fast track provisions.

Any changes to the approved product's indications, active ingredients, manufacture, or labeling require submission of a supplemental NDA (SNDA) for agency approval. Also, adverse drug reports are required by the agency. All reports must be reviewed by the manufacturer promptly, and if found to be serious, life-threatening, or unexpected (not listed in the product labeling), the manufacturer is required to submit an alert report within 15 working days of receipt of the information. All adverse reactions thought not to be serious or unexpected must be reported quarterly for 3 years after the application is approved, and annually thereafter.[26]

Over-the-counter (OTC) regulations

The 1951 Durham-Humphrey Amendments of the FDCA specified three criteria to justify prescription-only status. If the compound is shown to be habit forming, requires a prescriber's supervision, or has an NDA-prescription only limitation, it will require a prescription. The principles used to establish OTC status (no prescription required) are margin of safety, method of use, benefit-to-risk ratio, and adequacy of labeling for self-medication. For example, injectable drugs may not be given OTC with certain exceptions such as insulin. OTC market entry is less restrictive than that for prescription drugs and does not require pre-market clearance. They pose many fewer safety hazards than prescription drugs because they are designed to alleviate symptoms rather than disease. Easier access far outweighs the risks of side effects that can be adequately addressed through proper labeling.

As previously discussed, OTC products underwent a review in 1972. Because checking the 300,000+ OTC drug products in existence at the time would have been virtually impossible, FDA created OTC Advisory Panels to go over the data based on some 26 therapeutic categories. OTC drugs were only examined by active ingredient within a therapeutic category. Inactive ingredients were only examined provided they were shown to be safe and suitable for the product and did not interfere with effectiveness and quality.

This review of active ingredients resulted in the promulgation of a regulation or a monograph, which was a recipe or set of guidelines applicable to all OTC products within a therapeutic category. OTC monographs were general and required that OTC products show general recognition of the safety and effectiveness of the active ingredient. OTC products did not fall under prescription status if their active ingredients (or combinations) were deemed by FDA to be generally recognized as safe and effective (GRASE). The monograph system was a public system with a public comment component included after each phase of the process. Any products for which a final monograph was established remained on the market until one was determined.

There were four phases in the OTC monograph system. In Phase I, an expert panel was selected to review data for each active ingredient in each therapeutic category for safety, efficacy, and labeling. Their recommendations were made in the *Federal Register*. A public comment period of 30 to 60 days was permitted and supporting or contesting data were accepted for review. Then the panel reevaluated the data and published a "Proposed Monograph" in the *Federal Register* that publicly announced the conditions for which the panel believed the OTC products in a particular therapeutic class were GRASE and not misbranded. A "Tentative Final Monograph" was then developed and published stating the FDA position on the safety and efficacy of a particular ingredient within a therapeutic category and had acceptable labeling for indications, warnings, and directions for use. Active ingredients were deemed: Category I, GRASE for claimed therapeutic indications and not misbranded; Category II, not-GRASE and/or misbranded; Category III, insufficient data for determination.

After public comment, the final monograph was established and published with the FDA final criteria for which all drug products in a therapeutic class become GRASE and not misbranded. Following the effective date of the final monograph, all covered drug products that fail to conform to FDA requirements are considered misbranded and/or an unapproved new drug.[27]

However, since the monograph panels are no longer convened, many current products were switched from prescription status. A company that wishes to make this switch and offer a product to the U.S. marketplace can submit an amendment to a monograph to FDA which will act as the sole reviewer. The company may also file an SNDA provided that it has 3 years of marketing it as a prescription product, can demonstrate a relative high use during that period, and can validate that the product has a mild profile of adverse reactions. The last method involves a "Citizens Petition" which is rarely used.[27]

Regulating marketing

FDA has jurisdiction over prescription drug advertising and promotion. The basis for these regulations lies within the 1962 Kefauver-Harris Amendments. Essentially, any promotional information, in any form, must be truthful, fairly balanced, and fully disclosed. FDA views this information as either advertising or labeling. Advertising includes all traditional outlets in which a company places an ad. Labeling includes everything else including brochures, booklets, lectures, slide kits, letters to physicians, company-sponsored magazine articles, etc. All information must be truthful and not misleading. All material facts must be disclosed in a manner that is fairly balanced and accurate. If any of these requirements are violated, the product is considered misbranded for the indications for which it was approved under its NDA. FDA is also sensitive to the promotion of a product for off-label use. Off-label use occurs when a product is in some way presented in a manner that does not agree with or is not addressed in its approved labeling. Also, provisions of the Prescription Drug Marketing Act (PDMA) of 1987 apply. The Act prohibits company representatives from directly distributing or reselling prescription drug samples. Companies are required to establish a closed system of record keeping which will be able to track a sample from their control to that of a prescriber in order to prevent diversion. Prescribers are required to receive these samples and record and store them appropriately.[28]

Violations and enforcement

FDA has the power to enforce the regulations for any product as defined under the FDCA. It has the jurisdiction to inspect a manufacturer's premises and its records. After a facilities inspection, an agency inspector will issue an FDA Form 483s that describes observable violations. Response to the finding as described on this form must be made promptly. A warning letter may be used when the agency determines that one or more of a company's practices, products, or procedures are in violation of the FDCA. The FDA district has 15 days to issue a warning letter after an inspection. The company has 15 days in which to respond. If the company's response is satisfactory to the agency, no other action is warranted. If the response is not, the agency may request a recall of the violated products. However, FDA has no authority to force a company to recall a product, but it may force removal of a product through the initiation of a seizure.

Recalls fall into one of three classes. A Class I recall exists when there is a reasonable possibility that the use of a product will cause either serious adverse effects on health or death. Class II recalls are issued when the use of a product may cause temporary or medically reversible adverse effects on health, or where the probability of serious adverse effects on health is remote. A Class III recall occurs when the use of a product is not likely to cause adverse health consequences. Recalls are also categorized as consumer level, where the product is requested to be recalled from consumers' homes or control; a retail level, where the products are to be removed from retail shelves or control; and the wholesale level, where the product is to be removed from wholesale distribution. Companies who conduct recalls of their products are required to conduct effectiveness checks to determine the effectiveness of recalling the product from the marketplace.

If a company refuses to recall the product, FDA will seek an injunction against the company.[29] Issuance of an injunction is recommended to the Department of Justice (DOJ) by FDA. The DOJ takes the request to the federal court which issues an order that forbids a company from carrying out a particular illegal act, such as marketing a product FDA considers in violation of the FDCA. Companies can comply with the order and sign a consent agreement that specifies the changes required by FDA for the company to continue operations or companies can choose to litigate.

FDA may also initiate a seizure of violative products.[30] A seizure is ordered by the federal court in the district in which the products are located. The seizure order specifies products, their batch numbers, and any records determined by FDA as violative. The U.S. Marshals carry out this action. FDA institutes a seizure to prevent a company from selling, distributing, moving, or otherwise tampering with the product.

FDA may also debar individuals or firms from assisting or submitting an ANDA or directly providing services to any firm with an existing or pending drug product application. Debarment may last for up to 10 years.[31]

However, one of the more powerful deterrents that FDA uses is adverse publicity. The agency has no authority to require a company to advertise adverse publicity, but it does publish administrative actions against a company in any number of federal publications such as the *Federal Register*, the FDA Enforcement Report, the FDA Medical Bulletin, and the FDA Consumer.[32]

Summary

The laws and regulations that govern the U.S. pharmaceutical industry are both vast and complicated. Interpretation of the FDCA is in a constant state of flux. FDA is charged with this interpretation based on the rapid technological changes that are everyday occurrences within the industry. Many may suggest that more rapid drug approval places the citizenry in greater danger of adverse events. Others may reply that technology offers newer and more effective therapies for deadly diseases.

Historically, the U.S. Congress has passed laws governing medications based on reactions to crises. The Pure Food and Drug Act, the Food, Drug and Cosmetic Act, and the Price Competition and Patent Restoration Act are just a few. One hopes that this method of regulation will not continue as the norm. We can be proud of proactive legislation such as the Kefauver-Harris Amendments, the Orphan Drug Act, PDUFA, and FDAMA. These Acts have paved the way for meaningful change within the drug investigation process as we continue in our battle against disease. The U.S system of investigating new drugs is one that continues to have merit because it allows enough time to investigate benefit vs. risk. The American public can look forward to great advances from the industry and should be comfortable that FDA is watching.

Bibliography

1. Valentino, J., Practical uses for the USP: A legal perspective, in *Strauss's Federal Drug Laws and Examination Review*, 5th ed., Technomic Publishing, Lancaster, PA, 1999, p. 38.
2. Strauss, S., Food and drug administration: An overview, in *Strauss's Federal Drug Laws and Examination Review*, 5th ed., Technomic Publishing, Lancaster, PA, 1999, p. 323.
3. FDCA, Sec.21(g)(1).
4. Strauss, S., Food and drug administration: An overview, in *Strauss's Federal Drug Laws and Examination Review*, 5th ed., Technomic Publishing, Lancaster, PA, 1999, pp. 176, 186.
5. Pinna, K. and Pines, W., The Drugs/Biologics Approval Process, A Practical Guide to Food and Drug Law and Regulation, Food Drug Law Institute (FDLI), Washington, D.C., 1998, p. 96.
6. 21CFR58.
7. Pinna, K. and Pines, W., The Drugs/Biologics Approval Process, A Practical Guide to Food and Drug Law and Regulation, Food Drug Law Institute (FDLI), Washington, D.C., 1998, p. 98.
8. 21CFR56.
9. 21CFR50.
10. 21CFR314.
11. Pinna, K. and Pines, W., The Drugs/Biologics Approval Process, A Practical Guide to Food and Drug Law and Regulation, Food Drug Law Institute (FDLI), Washington, D.C., 1998, pp. 102–103.
12. Fed Reg, V.64(18), January 28, 1999.
13. Pinna, K. and Pines, W., The Drugs/Biologics Approval Process, A Practical Guide to Food and Drug Law and Regulation, Food Drug Law Institute (FDLI), Washington, D.C., 1998, p. 103.
14. Strauss, S., Food and drug administration: An overview, in *Strauss's Federal Drug Laws and Examination Review*, 5th ed., Technomic Publishing, Lancaster, PA, 1999, p. 280.
15. Food and Drug Administration Modernization Act of 1997, PL. 105, 1997.
16. 42USC, Sec. 262.
17. Form FDA 356h.
18. The Orphan Drug Act of 1982, PL 97-414.
19. The Orphan Drug Amendments of 1985, PL 99-91.
20. Pinna, K. and Pines, W., The Drugs/Biologics Approval Process, A Practical Guide to Food and Drug Law and Regulation, FDLI, Washington, D.C., 1998, p. 119.
21. USP/DI, Volume III, 13th Edition, Preface, v.
22. USP/DI, Volume III, 13th Edition p. I/7.
23. USP/DI, Volume III, 13th Edition p. I/9.
24. USP/DI, Volume III, 13th Edition p. I/10.
25. USP/DI, Volume III, 13th Edition p. I/12.

26. Pinna, K. and Pines, W., The Drugs/Biologics Approval Process, A Practical Guide to Food and Drug Law and Regulation, Food Drug Law Institute (FDLI), Washington, D.C., 1998, p. 111.
27. Strauss, S., Food and drug administration: An overview, in *Strauss's Federal Drug Laws and Examination Review*, 5th ed., Technomic Publishing, Lancaster, PA, 1999, p. 285
28. 21USC301, et seq.
29. 21USC302, et seq.
30. 21USC304, et seq.
31. Fundamentals of Regulatory Affairs, Regulatory Affairs Professions Society, 1999, p. 199.
32. Fundamentals of Regulatory Affairs, Regulatory Affairs Professions Society, 1999, p. 200.

chapter three

Federal laws and regulations governing pharmacy, pharmacists, and prescriptions

A comprehensive overview

The basis for all practice-oriented drug laws and regulations stems from the federal Controlled Substances Act (CSA of 1970) (21USC.801, et seq.). The Act, also known as Title II, was part of a much larger piece of legislation, the Comprehensive Drug Abuse Prevention and Control Act of 1970 (PL91-513). The CSA was enacted to regulate the manufacturing, distribution, dispensing, and delivery of drugs or substances that are subject to, or have the potential for, abuse or physical or psychological dependence. These drugs are designated as "controlled substances" because they are controlled under the CSA.[1]

The CSA falls under the regulatory authority of the Drug Enforcement Administration (DEA), which controls access to regulated substances. This control is achieved through the federal registration of all persons in the legitimate chain of manufacture, distribution, or dispensing of controlled substances, except the ultimate user.[2] The ultimate user is defined as (1) the patient who is competent to use these drugs as prescribed by a practitioner, or (2) the patient's caregiver who administers them to an incompetent patient, i.e., the parent of a sick child.[3] All healthcare providers who deal with the issue of pain management through the use of controlled substances are subject to the CSA as well as those drug control laws of the state in which they are licensed and practicing, unless such practice is exclusively in a federal facility, e.g., a Veterans Administration (VA) Hospital.[2]

The CSA empowers the DEA to register all persons, businesses, and institutions that would conduct any activity that would involve controlled substances by issuing them a registration number, the DEA number. A DEA registration must be renewed tri-annually.[4] In addition, the CSA established a closed-system of record-keeping provisions that control and track the flow of controlled substances through the healthcare system. For example, if a registrant, one who has been issued a DEA registration, wishes to order a controlled substance from a wholesaler or manufacturer, some very specific record-keeping provisions exist depending on how the drugs ordered are categorized or "scheduled."[5] All registrants who order, fulfill an order, store, distribute, or dispense a controlled substance must report this activity to DEA and maintain their own records for a period of 2 years.

The CSA places medicinal substances in schedules (or classes) in descending order based on their potential for abuse, psychological or physiological dependence, and their medical use. These substances include narcotics, amphetamines, and barbiturates and are denoted by a "C" and a roman numeral in the regulations and literature and on manufacturers' containers. Scheduling provisions also include prescription-dispensing limitations. There are five schedules of drugs as described by the CSA.

Much of what appears in the CSA also appears in state acts and regulations with some additional and more stringent modifications. For example, in Massachusetts, prescriptions issued for medications listed in Schedule II must be filled by a pharmacy within 5 days after the date on which it was issued.[6] Also, drugs listed in Schedule II or III are only fillable for a 30-day supply on any single filling.*[7,8] In addition, Massachusetts considers any prescription drug product not included in a federal schedule to be designated as Schedule VI.[9] Therefore, in Massachusetts, a patient's antihypertensive medication or prescription eye drops are considered to be controlled substances.

Federal vs. state laws and regulations

Each state has enacted various laws and regulations and has a counterpart to a federal administrative agency that controls the manufacture, distribution, and sale of drugs within the state and regulates the practice of healthcare professionals. Because one state's drug control laws may vary greatly from federal laws, certain basic principles must be followed by health professionals in order to comply. Fink et al.[10] suggest the following:

1. Health professionals are responsible for the same degree for compliance of both federal and state laws and regulations that govern their practices.
2. A state drug control law or regulation may be more stringent than its federal counterpart.

---

* Massachusetts law limits the filling of prescriptions for Schedule II drugs for up to a 30-day supply. However, dextro-amphetamine and methylphenidate are the exceptions and fillable in Massachusetts for up to a 60-day supply on any single filling.

3. Health professionals must comply with a state drug control law or regulation when it is stricter than federal law or no similar prohibition or requirement exists under federal law.
4. If a federal drug control law or regulation is more stringent than the comparable state law or regulation, the federal regulation must be followed.

Generally, most heathcare professionals do not make meaningful distinctions between federal and state laws and regulations to any great degree in their day-to-day practices. There simply would be little practical value in doing so. However, federal laws and regulations are the templates that all state regulatory agencies and their licencees must follow.

Prescription basics

Federal laws and regulations as well as those of many states require that prescriptions be complete with all requisite information (Figure 3.1). Prescriptions must be written in ink, in indelible pencil, or typewritten. Information may be entered onto a prescription by a designee, called an agent, of the prescriber or by a pharmacist when clarification is needed. The only information required in the prescriber's own handwriting is his or her personal signature. Federal law also allows Schedules III–V prescriptions to be orally and routinely telephoned into pharmacies from prescribers or their agents; pharmacists are required to record the name of that person onto that prescription.[11] These oral prescriptions must then be augmented by a written hardcopy within 7 days of its issuance. This hardcopy backup is the responsibility of the prescriber. Pharmacists who do not receive it are required to report this information to the DEA.

As alluded to previously, federal law categorizes prescription medications into schedules based on their abuse potential. As a result, these drugs need to be handled by prescribers and pharmacists in some very specific ways. Schedule II controlled substances are generally used for moderate to severe pain and have the most restrictions. Prescriptions written for medications listed in Schedule II are nonrefillable and require a written prescription only.[12]

Prescriptions for Schedule II controlled substances may be partially filled for quantities less than those prescribed because the pharmacy is out-of-stock or a patient requests less provided that the pharmacy dispenses the remainder to the patient within 72 hours. If unable to do so, the prescription becomes void for further quantity and the prescriber is so informed. Pharmacists may dispense partial quantities of Schedule II medications to patients in long-term care facilities (LTCF) or who are terminally ill for up to 60 days from the original date of the prescription's issuance. The dispensing pharmacist must record that the patient is in an LTCF or is terminally ill along with the date of dispensing, quantity dispensed, and remaining amount, with the dispensing pharmacist's signature on the back of the prescription.[13]

Schedule II medications also have restrictions on oral or telephone transmissions. The CSA allows prescribers to call pharmacies and orally transmit prescriptions for Schedule IIs only in an emergency situation. An "Emergency Situation" under the Controlled Substance Act means that immediate administration of the controlled substance is necessary for the proper treatment of the intended ultimate user; no appropriate alternative treatment is available, including administration of a drug that is not a controlled substance under Schedule II of the Act; and it is not reasonably possible for the prescribing physician to provide a written prescription to be presented to the person dispensing the substance prior to dispensing.

In case of an emergency situation, a pharmacist may dispense a Schedule II controlled substance upon receiving the orally transmitted authorization of a prescribing practitioner, provided that the quantity prescribed and dispensed is limited to the amount adequate to treat the patient during the emergency period. The prescribing practitioner must then provide a written prescription for the emergency quantity prescribed to be delivered or postmarked to the dispensing pharmacist within 7 days after authorizing an emergency oral prescription. In addition, the prescription shall have written on its face: "Authorization for Emergency Dispensing." Upon receipt of the written prescription, the dispensing pharmacist must attach the written prescription to the oral one. If the prescribing practitioner fails to deliver a written prescription within 7 days, the pharmacist shall notify the nearest office of the DEA.

The regulations for emergency situations can be cumbersome for home infusion pharmacies and hospice and long-term care pharmacies. Frequent dosage modifications of parenteral or controlled-release narcotic substances for patients who require these services can place pharmacies and prescribers at a regulatory disadvantage because the pharmacy has to enforce the existing regulations. However, DEA has provided an easier mechanism for handling prescriptions for CII pain medications. In May 1994, DEA issued a rule that allows controlled-substance prescription orders to be transmitted from a prescriber to a dispensing pharmacy by facsimile.* The rule covers all controlled-substance prescriptions. Of interest to our discussion, DEA allows pharmacies to receive facsimile prescriptions for intravenous pain therapy and retains them as the original prescription thereby substantially reducing the need for oral emergency prescriptions in these settings. One must note that these rules do not apply to oral dosage forms.

Prescriptions written for Schedules III and IV drugs have somewhat less stringent regulations attached to them. They are refillable up to five times if so authorized, or 6 months from their date of issue, whichever terminates first, and, when filled with a partial quantity, must have the quantity recorded on the back of the prescription along with the date of refilling and

---

* *Federal Register*, May 19, 1994.

the initials of the dispensing pharmacist.[15] Prescriptions written for Schedule V substances are also refillable; however, the number of refills is not set by law and the authorized number of refills depends on good professional judgment by the prescriber and the pharmacist.[11]

Pharmacists and prescribers are also co-liable for prescriptions written in err or with obvious problems. This is called "Corresponding Responsibility."[16] A prescription for a controlled substance must be issued in good faith and for a legitimate medical purpose by a practitioner in the usual course of his or her professional practice; likewise, pharmacists have the corresponding responsibility to ensure that the prescription is issued and dispensed in good faith for a legitimate medical purpose by a practitioner acting in the usual course of his or her practice. For example, if a pharmacist receives a prescription written by a radiologist for her child, what must the pharmacist do to protect herself from any corresponding responsibility? Radiologists are medical doctors with a specialty. However, this specialty does not preclude that person from prescribing medication outside his or her specialty provided that the prescription is written in good faith, for a legitimate medical purpose, and in the usual course of medical practice. If the radiologist conducted all of the medically required tests to reach a diagnosis and generated a patient record, thereby establishing a physician–patient relationship, the prescription would be fillable under federal law. Pharmacists will question prescriptions such as this to protect themselves and their patients.

Summary of Federal Prescription Filling Laws and Regulations

Schedule	CI	CII	CIII	CIV	CV
Examples	Heroin/PCP High abuse potential and no accepted medical use in the United States	Morphine Percodan Amphetamines Barbiturates	APAP/codeine or other tablets/ capsules with codeine Anabolic steroids	Diazepam Phenobarbital Meprobamate Propoxyphene	Cough syrups/ codeine Lomotil
Time valid for filling	None	None or state mandate	180 days from date of issue	180 days from date of issue	None
Max days supply per fill	None	None or state mandate	180 days	180 days	None
Max refills	None	No refills allowed	5 refills	5 refills	None
Oral Rx allowed	None	Emergency only	Yes	Yes	Yes

Product selection

Product selection is another issue that causes pharmacists and prescribers much anguish. Product selection may be divided into two categories: (1) the substitution of products that are pharmaceutically equivalent and are bioequivalent, i.e., a brand-name product and a generic copy; and (2) the substitution of chemically dissimilar products that are in the same therapeutic class, i.e., two therapeutic moieties that treat the same medical condition.

The substitution of products with the same active ingredients is well defined in the regulations of many states. Generally, the list of substitutable products used by pharmacists and sanctioned by the states stems from a federal publication published since 1979 by FDA called, "Approved Drug Products with Therapeutic Equivalence Evaluations." This document is prepared as a guide for healthcare professionals in making product selection decisions. It lists marketed drug products that are considered by FDA to be safe and effective and provides information on therapeutic equivalence evaluations for approved multisource prescription drug products.[17] The Orange Book is republished by the USP in the third volume of the set entitled "USP/Dispensing Information" (USP/DI). As new drug products are approved or evaluated, they appear in the Orange Book and USP/DI in the form of monthly supplements and annual publications.

Drug products with an A rating are determined by FDA to be therapeutically equivalent and may be substituted. Drug products with B ratings are not considered by FDA to be therapeutically equivalent and may not be substituted. However, because the Orange Book is merely a guide to therapeutic equivalence, state agencies, such the Massachusetts Department of Public Health, have the option of deciding to allow some B-rated products to be substituted if the determination can be made that bioequivalence is not essential.[22] The only practical way for health professionals to know whether a drug is listed is to consult the Orange Book and any other references available in the home state. Please refer to the information in Chapter 2 on Abbreviated New Drug Application (ANDA) for a review of the criteria for generic drugs.

Currently, some 13 states require pharmacists to substitute one product for another depending on how a prescription is written. This is called mandatory substitution and leaves pharmacists little choice but to comply. Thirty-nine states allow a more permissive substitution where patients may be asked if they wish to receive a substitutable product based on cost or pharmacist suggestion. In addition, many states have a positive formulary allowing pharmacists to dispense only substitutable products from an established list of drugs. Others have a negative formulary that allows pharmacists to substitute any product they wish provided it *does not* appear on the established list.[23]

The substitution of products within a therapeutic category in which two therapeutic moieties can be used alternatively to treat the same medical condition may also be an issue of great angst. Hospital pharmacy and therapeutics committees as well as managed care organizations (MCOs) and others who control formularies are constantly searching for the most therapeutic and cost-effective medications to treat medical problems. At issue are the great depth and breadth of medications available. One would have many optimal choices were it not for product cost. Therefore, medication management decision makers must choose which medications will be used for particular medical conditions or patients based on overall clinical effectiveness and cost.

The prescription

```
                        Name of Practitioner
                        Address of Practitioner


    Date of Issue
    DEA Registration Number


    Name of Patient (Unless Veterinary)
    Address of Patient


    Rx              Name/Strength/Dosage of Medication/Quantity


                    Sig:    Directions for use and any cautionary statements


                    Number of Times to Be Refilled.


                        Signature of Prescriber
```

Figure 3.1 The prescription.

Let us begin at the beginning. A prescription is considered complete when the following information is included on its face:

1. Date of issue
2. Name, address of practitioner
3. Controlled substance registration number
4. Name of patient
5. Address of patient
6. Name, strength, dose, and quantity of controlled substances
7. Directions for use and any cautionary statements required
8. Number of times to be refilled
9. Signature of prescriber

Prescriptions must be written in ink, indelible pencil, or typewritten. They may be prepared by a physician's secretary or agent, but must be manually signed by the physician who issues the order. In addition, prescriptions may only be issued by a physician, dentist, podiatrist, veterinarian, or other registered practitioners who are authorized by the jurisdiction in which they are licensed to practice to prescribe controlled substances.

Oral prescriptions

A prescription may be transmitted both orally and routinely in Schedules III–V from any agent of the prescriber to the registered pharmacist. The pharmacist must place the name of the person who transmitted the prescription on the face of the oral prescription.

Prescriptions may be filled in a community pharmacy when written by interns, residents, and foreign physicians in a hospital who have been assigned a suffix to the institutional DEA number.

Schedules III and IV

Prescriptions written for Schedules III and IV are refillable up to five times or 6 months from the date of issue, whichever terminates first if so authorized. The initials of the dispensing pharmacist and the quantity dispensed must appear on the back of the prescription when filling a partial quantity. All partial dispensing must be done within 6 months of the issuance of the original prescription.

Schedule V

Prescriptions written for Schedule V are refillable; however, the number of refills is not set by law and the authorized number of refills depends on good professional judgment by both the prescriber and the pharmacist.

Schedule V controlled substances sold OTC

Regulations allow a pharmacist to sell Schedule V, non-narcotic, narcotic, and non-legend preparations without a prescription with proper record keeping (excepted compounds). Pharmacists may not sell more than 240 ml or 48 solid dosage units of opium-containing substances, or 120 ml or 24 solid dosage units of non-opium-containing controlled substances may be dispensed within a 48-hour period. The purchaser must be known to the pharmacist or provide identification to the pharmacist and must be at least 18 years of age at the time of sale. These preparations generally contain opium derivatives for the control of coughs or diarrhea.

The pharmacy must maintain a bound book to record the dispensing of Schedule V substances for a period of 2 years and include the following information:

1. Name and address of purchaser
2. Name and quantity of controlled substance
3. Date of sale
4. Initials or name of dispensing pharmacist

Transferring prescriptions

The transfer of existing, filled prescriptions is allowable under federal law for prescription drugs in Schedules III through V. The transfer may be conducted one time only. The transfer rule only applies in conjunction with state pharmacy law. Individual states may have more stringent requirements.

Schedule II controlled substances

Prescriptions written for Schedule II controlled substances must be treated to a somewhat different standard than those in other schedules. The basic regulations are as follows:

1. CII prescriptions are nonrefillable.
2. A written prescription is required.
3. Prescriptions are valid for 60 days from their date of issuance for patients in a long-term care facility (LTCF) or who are medically diagnosed to be terminally ill.
4. Drug must be secured in a locked and substantially constructed cabinet or dispersed throughout the stock of non-controlled substances in such a manner as to obstruct their theft or diversion.

Oral emergency prescriptions for Schedule II

Prescriptions may be called into a pharmacy by a prescriber in only certain, well-defined circumstances termed "emergency situations." An emergency situation under the Controlled Substance Act means:

1. Immediate administration of the controlled substance is necessary for the proper treatment for the intended ultimate user.
2. No appropriate alternative treatment is available, including administration of a drug that is not a controlled substance under Schedule II of the Act.
3. It is not reasonably possible for the prescribing physician to provide a written prescription to be presented to the person dispensing the substance prior to dispensing.

In the case of an emergency situation a pharmacist may only dispense enough medication to carry the patient through the emergency or until the patient can access the prescriber. The pharmacist must copy the information in proper form onto a prescription blank and write the words, "EMERGENCY AUTHORIZATION" on its face. A prescribing physician is required to mail or hand-deliver a written, hard-copy prescription to the dispensing pharmacy to cover the oral emergency supply of medication within 7 days. Pharmacists are required to attach this hard copy to the oral copy on receipt. If the pharmacist does not receive the hard-copy backup prescription from the physician within the 7-day period as required by federal law and regulation, the pharmacist then is required to contact DEA and report the missing prescription.

Methadone

Prescriptions for methadone are valid provided that the drug is used as an analgesic. They are not valid through the typical retail pharmacy distribution channels for the purposes of detoxification or maintenance therapy for drug addiction. However, when written by a physician for an addicted patient, a single-day quantity for 3 consecutive days may be prescribed for the purposes of admitting that addicted person to an appropriately licensed treatment program.

Partial filling

Prescriptions partially filled for Schedule II controlled substances require:

1. The quantity filled to be noted on the face of the prescription.
2. The remainder be filled within 72 hours.
3. Beyond 72 hours the prescription becomes void for further quantity and the prescriber so informed.
4. Long-term care facilities (LTCF) and "Terminally Ill" patients only.
    a. Pharmacist must record that the patient is in a LTCF or is terminally ill.
    b. Pharmacist must record the date, quantity dispensed *and* remaining, and the initials or signature of the dispensing pharmacist on the back of the prescription.

Electronically transmitted/faxed prescriptions

Prescriptions or drug orders for controlled substances listed in Schedules III–V may be routinely transmitted by facsimile machine, computer modem, or other similar electronic device directly from an authorized prescribing practitioner or his or her expressly authorized agent to a pharmacy or pharmacy department of the patient's choice. The faxed copy may be retained as the hard-copy original and will be considered compliant with all federal regulations provided it contains all information as required under federal laws and regulations. This electronically transmitted or faxed prescription may be filed with other prescriptions in the customary fashion.

Schedule II faxed prescriptions

Prescriptions faxed to pharmacies for medications listed in Schedule II must be treated somewhat differently based on where the patient resides. If the patient is ambulatory or resides at home, the original, signed prescription shall be presented to the dispensing pharmacist before the electronically transmitted filled prescription is released to the patient.

However, federal law allows two exceptions to this rule:

1. *Intravenous pain therapy, or home or hospice infusion.* The original prescription need not be sent to the pharmacy either before or after the medication is delivered to a patient's home. The faxed copy is considered to be the original prescription and must be retained as such.
2. *Long-term care facilities.* Faxed prescriptions for patients in long-term care facilities are considered to be the original written prescription order.

U.S. postal regulations

U.S. Postal Regulations allow the mailing of any filled prescription containing a narcotic of any quantity or federal schedule to patients. When mailing controlled substances, two rules must be followed:

1. The inner container must be marked, sealed, and labeled with the name and address of the practitioner, or the name and address of the pharmacy or other person dispensing the prescription, and the prescription number.
2. The outside wrapper or container must be plain with no markings of any kind that would indicate the contents contained within.

Corresponding responsibility

A prescription for a controlled substance must be issued in good faith and for a legitimate medical purpose by a practitioner in the usual course of his or her professional practice; likewise, pharmacists have the corresponding responsibility to ensure that the prescription is issued and dispensed in good faith for a legitimate medical purpose by a practitioner acting in the usual course of his or her practice. However, physicians may write prescriptions for any medication, regardless of practice specialty, providing a proper diagnosis and a physician–patient relationship have been established.

Prescription labeling

The prescription label must be affixed to a container and must contain the following information:

1. Pharmacy name, address, and telephone number
2. Assigned serial number
3. Date of initial dispensing
4. Name of patient
5. Name of prescriber

6. Directions for use and any cautionary statements
7. Federal controlled substances warning label or "transfer label" for Schedules II, III, and IV controlled substance

A controlled substance warning label, also known as the "Federal Transfer Label," must be affixed to prescription containers of any drug listed in Schedules II–IV. The label reads as follows:

> CAUTION: Federal law prohibits the transfer of this drug to any person other than the patient for whom it was prescribed.

Expiration or beyond-use dates

Expiration dates listed on a manufacturer's stock container are set based on appropriate stability data that would support length of shelf life. However, many states require some form of expiration dating on prescription labels. Most use the standards as described by the United States Pharmacopeia. USP 21 states:

> Unless otherwise specified in the individual monograph, such beyond-use date (expiration date) shall be not later than the expiration date on the manufacturer's container, or one year from the date from when the drug is dispensed, whichever is earlier.

However, this standard applies only to those prescriptions dispensed to patients in ambulatory or community settings. Medications dispensed to patients in long-term care settings or similar institutions or those repackaged into unit dose packaging or unit of use containers must use the expiration date, which is either 6 months from the date of dispensing, or represents 25% of the time remaining on the manufacturer's container, whichever is earlier.

In addition, the USP specifies that the expiration date for insulin products is 24 months from their date of manufacture. OTC drug products are exempt from expiration dating if they are stable for at least 3 years, have no dosing limitations, and are safe and suitable for frequent and prolonged use. Some examples of these products include toothpaste and medicated shampoo.

Safety closures and containers

In accordance with the Poison Prevention Packaging Act of 1970, child-resistant closures must be used on prescription containers unless the prescription is for an exempt drug, e.g., sublingual nitroglycerin, cholestyramine powder, unit dose or effervescent potassium supplements, erythromycin ethylsuccinate preparations, and oral contraceptives packaged in mnemonic packages.

Patients may authorize conventional, easy-to-open packaging for good reason and even issue a blanket waiver for prescription containers. This authorization may be in writing or oral. A physician may *not* issue a blanket waiver for dispensing in conventional, easy-to-open packaging; the order must be on each prescription.

In addition, refills of prescriptions dispensed in plastic containers require new containers to ensure that the locking mechanism does not become worn and ineffective through constant use. Refills of prescriptions dispensed in glass containers require that only the caps be replaced.

The pharmacy

Every pharmacy must be registered with DEA and receive a certificate of registration to distribute or dispense controlled substances; each pharmacy has its own DEA Registration Number. These certificates of registration must be renewed every 3 years. Every pharmacy registrant must keep and maintain an accurate record of each controlled substance received. Dated invoices for controlled substances in Schedules III, IV, and V will constitute complete records for these drugs. Copy 3 of DEA Form-222, discussed later, will constitute complete records for the receipt of Schedule II controlled substances. DEA requires every registrant who changes his or her business address to notify it and receive approval prior to moving. Registrants may keep records at a location other than the registered location by notifying the nearest DEA office. Unless this request denied, registrants may transfer records 14 days after notification.

Record keeping

One of the primary tasks of the pharmacy registrant is record keeping. DEA as well as state agencies have specific requirements that all DEA registrants must follow. All records of receipt and distribution of controlled substances must be kept at the site for 2 years. For example, all DEA registrants must keep a complete and accurate inventory of all federally controlled substances. The requirements are as follows.

Inventory requirements

An initial inventory must be taken as soon as controlled substance activities are engaged. If no controlled substances are on hand, a zero inventory should be recorded. The initial inventory must contain the name, address, DEA number of the registrant, the date and time of the inventory, the signature of the person taking the inventory, as well as the name of the medication,

Common Controlled Substances (Representative Examples)

SCHEDULE I
LSD
Methaqualone
Diacetylmorphine (Heroin)
Mescaline
Psilocybin
Marijuana

SCHEDULE II
Narcotics
Cocaine
Codeine
Fentanyl (Duragesic)
Hydromorphone (Dilaudid)
Meperidine (Demerol)
Methadone (Dolophine)
Morphine (MS Contin)
Opium Tinc/Deodorized
Oxycodone-ASA (Percodan)
Oxycodone-APAP (Percocet, Tylox)
Tetrahydrocannabinol (Marinol)

Barbiturates
Amobarbital (Amytal)
Pentobarbital (Nembutal)
Secobarbital (Seconal)

Amphetamines
Dextroamphetamine (Dexedrine)
Methylphenidate (Ritalin)

SCHEDULE III
Anabolic Steroids
APAP-Codeine (Tylenol with Codeine)
ASA-Codeine (Empirin with Codeine)
Butalbital-ASA-Caffeine (Fiorinal)
Hycodan Syrup
Hycomine Syrup
Hydrocodone-APAP (Vicodin)
Opium Tinc/Camphorated (Paregoric)
Tussionex Suspension

SCHEDULE IV
Anti-Anxiety Agents
Alprazolam (Xanax)
Chlordiazepoxide (Librium)
Clonazepam (Klonopin)
Clorazepate Dipotassium (Tranxene)
Diazepam (Valium)
Lorazepam (Ativan)
Meprobamate (Equanil)
Oxazepam (Serax)

Sleep Inducers
Chloral Hydrate (Noctec)
Flurazepam (Dalmane)
Temazepam (Restoril)

Anorectics
Diethylpropion (Tepanil/Tenuate)
Phentermine Resin (Ionamin)
Phentermine HCL (Fastin)

Narcotics
Propoxyphene HCL (Darvon)
Propoxyphene Napsylate with APAP (Darvocet)
Pentazocine with Naloxone (Talwin-Nx)

Miscellaneous
Phenobarbital

SCHEDULE V
Cough syrups with Codeine
Robitussin AC
Phergan with Codeine Elixir

Anti-diarrheals
Diphenoxylate with Atropine (Lomotil)

dosage form, dosage, and quantity on hand. Then, once every 2 years following the date of the original inventory, a biennial inventory must be taken of all federally controlled substances (CII–V). This biennial inventory may be taken on any date with the 2-year period. DEA requires exact counting of all medications listed in Schedule II. Medications listed in Schedules III,

IV, and V may be estimated provided the original package size was less that 1000 solid dosage units. If the original package size is 1000 solid dosage units or greater, an exact count must be made. Schedule II inventories must be kept separately from all other records of controlled substances. All controlled substance inventory records must be kept at the inventory location for a period of 2 years.

Federal regulation allows pharmacists to file filled prescriptions in one of three ways. Pharmacy practitioners should be cautioned that the laws and regulations of their home state may differ. The federal requirement is as follows:

1. Pharmacists may keep two files, one containing Schedule IIs and the other containing Schedules III, IV, V and nonscheduled drugs. If this method is chosen, all federally controlled substances, i.e., III, IV, and V, must be stamped with a large red "C," no less than 1 in. high, in the lower right-hand corner to make those prescriptions readily retrievable.
2. Pharmacists may also keep two files: (1) one for all federally controlled substances, marking those prescriptions for Schedules III, IV, and V with a large red "C," and (2) one containing non-controlled substances.
3. The third method of filing prescriptions includes three separate files: one file for Schedule IIs, one file for Schedules III, IV, and V, and one file for non-controlled substances.

Computerized prescription processing systems

Federal laws and regulations permit much of its record-keeping requirement to be accomplished via computerized prescription processing systems. A pharmacy may use such a system for the storage and retrieval of prescription information provided it can immediately retrieve information by either CRT display or hard-copy printout for prescriptions currently being filled. The information necessary for retrieval must include, but is not be limited to:

1. Date of issuance
2. Original prescription number
3. Name and address of patient
4. Physician's name and DEA number
5. Name, strength, dosage form, and quantity of controlled substance
6. Total number of refills authorized by the physician

The system must provide a refill history by CRT or hard-copy for controlled substances that have been refilled during the past 6 months. Pharmacies that use a computerized prescription processing system must print a hard-copy or receive a hard-copy from a central processor within 72 hours of dispensing. Pharmacists who dispense these prescriptions must then verify that the information on the hard-copy is correct and then sign and date that printout. A hard-copy printout or other documentation must be stored in a separate file for a period of 2 years.

DEA forms

Form 222

All Schedule I and II drugs purchased to stock a pharmacy or other registered location must be ordered using DEA Form-222. In addition, pharmacists wishing to borrow or transfer (from registrant to registrant) Schedule II controlled substances from other pharmacies may do so only by using a DEA Form-222. The form is in triplicate and may be signed by the registrant or any person who has written authorization to do so, e.g., Power of Attorney. Power of Attorney refers to any individual or individuals authorized by the pharmacy to sign and obtain DEA-222 order forms on behalf of the pharmacy. These individuals do not necessarily need to be registered pharmacists.

Each form contains ten lines on which to write the CII medication to be ordered. One line on the order form should be used to describe one item; if two lines are used for the same item, they count as only one line. These forms must submitted to the supplier error free. Therefore, voiding a line on the order form due to an error is not permitted and the entire form should be voided. When complete, the person ordering the medication must separate the third copy of the form and retain it in the pharmacy. Upon receipt of the drugs, the person who has ordered them, or any other authorized person, must fill out the last two columns of the store's copy with quantity and date.

Form 106

Loss of controlled substances (federal Schedules II–V) must be reported to the district DEA office on DEA Form-106. If the pharmacy is involved in a robbery or if a significant shortage of controlled substances is detected, after reporting to the local police department, a DEA Form-106 should be filled out in triplicate. Two copies must be sent to the regional DEA office as soon as possible; one copy must be kept on file by the pharmacy.

The information on DEA Form-106 should contain:

1. Name and address of the firm
2. DEA registration number
3. Date of theft
4. Local police department notified
5. Type of theft (robbery, break-in, etc.)
6. A listing of any symbols or cost codes used by the pharmacy, if any
7. A listing of any missing controlled substances

Form 41

Used for the destruction of controlled substances. DEA should be contacted for instructions when there is a need to destroy outdated, damaged, or otherwise unusable controlled substances. DEA has authorized private companies to administrate controlled substances destruction. The agency should be contacted for further information.

Miscellaneous

Patient Package Inserts (PPIs) are required by FDA regulation to be provided to the patient when dispensing certain drugs. PPIs must be given to the patient on the initial dispensing and on refills if so requested.

All of the following are drugs that must be dispensed with a PPI:

1. Isoproterenol inhalation products
2. Oral contraceptives
3. Estrogen/progestogen-containing drug products
4. Intrauterine devices
5. Progestational drug products
6. Accutane R

A prescription for an approved drug may be filled for an unapproved use provided that the prescriber:

1. Is well informed about the drug prescribed
2. Bases such use on firm scientific rationale or sound medical evidence
3. Maintains adequate records of drug use and effect

Bibliography

1. Fink, J.L., Marquardt, K.W., and Simonsmeir, L.M., *Pharmacy Law Digest*, 26th ed., Facts and Comparisons, Inc., St. Louis, MO, Nov. 1995, p. CS-1.
2. Fink, J.L., Marquardt, K.W., and Simonsmeir, L.M., *Pharmacy Law Digest*, 26th ed., Facts and Comparisons, Inc., St. Louis, MO, Nov. 1995, p. CS-2.
3. Massachusetts General Law, Ch.94c, Sec. 1, Definitions.
4. 21CFR1301.21.
5. 21CFR1305 et seq.
6. Massachusetts General Law, Ch.94c, Sec.23(b).
7. Massachusetts General Law, Ch.94c, Sec.23(b)(d).
8. Massachusetts General Law, Ch.94C, Sec. 23(d).
9. Massachusetts General Law, Ch.94c, Sec.2(a).
10. Fink, J.L., Marquardt, K.W., and Simonsmeir, L.M., *Pharmacy Law Digest*, 26th ed., Facts and Comparisons, Inc., St. Louis, MO, Nov. 1995, p. CS-4.
11. 21CFR1306.21.
12. 21CFR1306.11.

13. 21CFR1306.13.
14. Federal Register, May 19, 1994.
15. 21CFR1306.22.
16. 21CFR1306.04.
17. USP/DI, Volume III, 13th Edition, Preface, v.
18. USP/DI, p.I/7.
19. USP/DI, p.I/9.
20. USP/DI, p.I/10.
21. USP/DI, p.I/12.
22. 105CMR720.050(b).
23. NABP Survey of Pharmacy Law, p. 50. (As of 2000.)

chapter four

DEA registration

Who may be issued a DEA registration?

A DEA registration may be issued to a host of qualified healthcare and nonhealthcare professionals as needed to treat patients, dispense controlled substances, conduct research, manufacture, repackage, wholesale, or teach. As previously discussed, a DEA registration may be issued to physicians, dentists, podiatrists, veterinarians, mid-level practitioners, or other registered practitioners who are authorized to prescribe controlled substances by the jurisdiction in which he or she is licensed to practice and who are registered with DEA or exempted from registration such as those who practice for the U.S. Public Health Service and/or Bureau of Prison physicians.[1] These registrations must be renewed tri-annually (every 3 years).

DEA registration numbers

A DEA registration number for a practitioner begins with either the letter "A" or "B." Registration numbers issued to mid-level practitioners begin with the letter M. The first letter of the registration number is followed by the first letter of the registrant's last name (e.g., J for Jones or S for Smith), and then a computer-generated sequence of seven numbers (such as MJ3614511).[1] The computer-generated sequence of seven numbers may be of benefit to pharmacists in their efforts to deter prescription fraud. The computer randomly generates the first six numbers and calculates the final number according to the following formula: add the sum of the numbers in the odd position to the sum of the numbers in the even position multiplied by 2. The second number in the final sum is called the "check digit" and is the last number in the sequence. For example, using MJ3614511, the letter "M" represents the practitioner as a mid-level prescriber. The letter "J" represents the first letter of the last name "Jones." The numbers are randomly generated and the final "check digit" is the number "1." The formula is as follows:

1st	2nd	3rd	4th	5th	6th	7th
odd	even	odd	even	odd	even	check
3	6	1	4	5	1	1

Odd position: $3 + 1 + 5 = 9$
Even position: $6 + 4 + 1 = 11 \times 2 = 22$
$22 + 9 = 31$ ("1" is the 7th or check digit)

Registration

Pharmacies seeking to become registered for the first time must request a DEA Form-224. Any pharmacy engaged in cooperative buying of controlled substances must also register as a distributor with the DEA. To obtain this registration, a pharmacy must meet distributor (wholesaler) security and record-keeping requirements. An affidavit system for expediting pharmacy applications may be used to obtain a DEA registration number for a new pharmacy or for transferring ownership of an existing pharmacy. Any time a pharmacy moves to a new physical location or the postal address changes at the same location, a new DEA certificate reflecting the new address must be obtained. It is the pharmacy's responsibility to notify DEA about a change of address before the effective date of the move. A written request for modification of registration should be sent to the DEA Registration Field Office responsible for the pharmacy's state. If the modification is approved, DEA will issue a new certificate of registration and, if requested, new Schedule II order forms (DEA Form-222). A Renewal Application for Registration (DEA Form-224a) will only be sent to the registered address on file with DEA. It cannot be forwarded.[1]

Transferring a pharmacy business

A registrant transferring a pharmacy business to another registrant[1] must notify the nearest DEA Registration Field Office at least 14 days before the date of the proposed transfer and provide the following information:

1. The name, address, and registration number of the registrant discontinuing business
2. The name, address, and registration number of the registrant acquiring the pharmacy
3. Whether the business activities will be continued at the location registered by the current business owner or moved to another location; if the latter, give the address of the new location

4. The date on which the controlled substances will be transferred to the person acquiring the pharmacy

On the day the controlled substances are transferred, a complete controlled substances inventory must be taken and a copy of the inventory must be included in the records of both the person transferring the business and the person acquiring the business.[1]

If the registrant acquiring the pharmacy owns at least one other pharmacy licensed in the same state as the pharmacy being transferred, the registrant may apply for a new DEA registration prior to the date of transfer. DEA will issue a registration that will authorize the registrant to obtain controlled substances at the time of transfer, but the registrant may not dispense controlled substances until the pharmacy has been issued a valid state pharmacy license.[1]

A DEA registration application for transferring ownership of an existing pharmacy can be expedited if the applicant includes an affidavit verifying that the pharmacy has been registered by the state licensing agency. The affidavit verifying the existence of the state license should be attached to the initial application for registration.[1]

Practitioners

A practitioner as defined above may be issued a DEA registration number which authorizes that practitioner to prescribe controlled substances to patients. However, the issuance of a DEA number does not permit all practitioners to write prescriptions for any patient ailment. As discussed in Chapter 3, to be valid a prescription for a controlled substance must be issued for a legitimate medical purpose by a practitioner acting in the usual course of sound professional practice. The practitioner is responsible for the proper prescribing and dispensing of controlled substances. However, a corresponding responsibility rests with the pharmacist who dispenses the prescription. An order for controlled substances which purports to be a valid prescription, but is not issued in the usual course of professional treatment or for legitimate and authorized research is not a valid prescription within the meaning and intent of the Controlled Substances Act (CSA). An individual who knowingly dispenses such a purported prescription, as well as the individual issuing it, will be subject to criminal and/or civil penalties and administrative sanctions. A prescription may not be issued in order for an individual practitioner to obtain a supply of controlled substances for the purpose of general dispensing to his or her patients. Therefore, a prescription written for office stock or "medical bag" use is not valid.[1]

This means a practitioner who prescribes for a "legitimate medical purpose" (defined as the use of the medication is for a medically acceptable course of treatment) and is acting in the "usual course of sound professional practice" (meaning the prescription is for an actual patient who has been diagnosed with a disease, condition, or symptom and has a medical record generated and is being treated for a medical condition that is within the usual treatment of that practitioner). Therefore, if the patient is being treated by a medical doctor who has studied all of the human organ systems, the practitioner's scope of medical practice and actions in the usual course of sound professional practice (making the proper diagnosis), the physician practitioner may prescribe a controlled substance for any medical condition that the patient presents. In other words, medical doctors do not have a restricted scope of professional practice. This is not the case for other categories of practitioners. For example, veterinarians are restricted in their usual course of sound professional practice to the treatment of diseases found in animals. Dentists similarly are restricted to treating diseases of teeth, gums, and the oral cavity.

Mid-level practitioners

Mid-level practitioners (MLPs) are registered and authorized by the DEA and the state in which they practice to dispense, administer, and prescribe controlled substances in the course of professional practice. Examples of MLPs include, but are not limited to, healthcare providers such as nurse practitioners, nurse midwives, nurse anesthetists, clinical nurse specialists, physician assistants, optometrists, ambulance services, animal shelters, veterinarian euthanasia technicians, and nursing homes and homeopathic physicians.[1]

MLPs may receive individual DEA registration granting controlled substance privileges. However, such registration is contingent upon authority granted by the state in which they are licensed. DEA registers MLPs whose states clearly authorize them to prescribe, dispense, and administer controlled substances listed in one or more schedules. The fact that an MLP has been issued a valid DEA registration number (beginning with the letter M) will be evidence that he or she is authorized to prescribe, dispense, and/or administer at least some controlled substances.

However, it will still be incumbent upon the pharmacist who fills the prescription to ensure that the MLP is prescribing within the parameters established by the state in which he or she practices. MLP authority to prescribe controlled substances varies greatly by state. Check with the state licensing or controlled substances authority to determine which MLP disciplines are authorized to prescribe controlled substances.[1]

Practitioner's use of a hospital's DEA registration number

An individual practitioner (e.g., intern, resident, staff physician, mid-level practitioner) who is an agent or employee of a hospital or other institution may, when acting in the usual course of business or employment, administer, dispense, or prescribe controlled substances under the registration of the hospital or other institution in which he or she is employed, provided that

1. The dispensing, administering, or prescribing is in the usual course of professional practice.
2. The practitioner is authorized to do so by the state in which he or she is practicing.
3. The hospital or institution has verified that the practitioner is permitted to dispense, administer, or prescribe controlled substances within the state.
4. The practitioner acts only within the scope of employment in the hospital or institution.

The hospital or institution will authorize the practitioner to dispense or prescribe under its registration and will assign a specific internal code number, with a suffix for each practitioner so authorized. For example, if Metropolitan Hospital's DEA registration number is BM1111119 and a visiting physician is granted practice privileges at that institution, the institution would issue the physician an internal code which is required to appear on all prescriptions written. That code would be included on the end of the DEA registration number for the hospital as a suffix, i.e., BM1111119-Q23.

A current list of internal codes and corresponding individual practitioners is to be kept by the hospital or other institution. This list is to be available at all times to other registrants and law enforcement agencies upon request for the purpose of verifying the authority of the prescribing individual practitioner. Pharmacists should contact the hospital or other institution for verification if they have any doubts in dispensing such a prescription.

Bibliography

1. Pharmacists Manual, Drug Enforcement Administration, Washington, D.C., March 2001, p. 41.

chapter five

A pharmacist's liability and the legal issues of OBRA '90 and patient counseling

Introduction

The passage of the Medicaid Prudent Pharmaceutical Purchasing Act (MPPPA) by the United States Congress in 1990 has created enormous upheaval to the traditional practice of community pharmacy as we knew it. The MPPPA was a small portion of the federal budget, the Omnibus Budget Reconciliation Act of 1990, and is more colloquially known as OBRA '90. In the years since its passage, pharmacists have been deluged with information regarding the effects of OBRA '90 on pharmacy practice by the professional press. This chapter examines some of the changes caused by the furor regarding the requirements of OBRA '90 that specify drug therapy review and counseling of patients

OBRA '90 requires that pharmacists must offer to counsel each individual patient or caregiver in at least the following ways:

1. The name and description of the medication
2. The route of administration, dosage, and dosage form
3. Special precautions for the preparation, administration, or use of the medication by the patient
4. Common severe side effects, adverse effects, interactions, and contra-indications that may be encountered
5. Techniques for self-monitoring therapy
6. Proper medication storage
7. Prescription refill information
8. Any action that should be taken in the event of a missed dose

OBRA '90 requires pharmacists to obtain, record, and maintain certain documentation regarding Medicaid patients which should include at least the following:

1. Name, address, telephone number, age, gender
2. Disease state(s)
3. Known allergies/drug reactions
4. Comprehensive list of medications
5. Any relevant medical devices
6. Pharmacist's comments relative to a patient's therapy

OBRA '90 had the potential to turn into a legal nightmare for community pharmacy practitioners. Much of the way community practice had to be rethought and reorganized was for reasons well beyond compliance with the law. The many-faceted issues associated with risk management and professional liability were in the forefront. It would be unconscionable for any member of the profession to believe that OBRA '90 and the subsequent laws and regulations enacted by states and their boards of pharmacy do not present a healthy complement of potentially litigious baggage.

OBRA '90 and its mandates require that pharmacists *"do* something." In doing that something, there is a responsibility to do it as required by law and in accordance with national practice standards. OBRA '90 offers the possibility of penalty when pharmacists do not do something, do it incorrectly, or do not do enough of that something. As an example, if a pharmacist counsels a patient about a medication and does not include some significant piece of information, either intentionally or not, there is the possibility of a lawsuit or administrative sanction. If this notion sounds confusing or vague, it should, because it is difficult to predict just what the legal ramifications will actually be. Though there have been some court cases, much of the activity around OBRA '90 and its patient counseling components has occurred at the state board of pharmacy level. Many who are involved with pharmacy practice and law still feel that the profession will need to wait and see what kinds of litigation arise since relying on decisions of past lawsuits against pharmacists may not be very helpful.

There are a few key legal cases pertaining to pharmacists that serve to demonstrate the dilemma faced by the courts regarding what pharmacists can or should do. In one of the earliest cases, *Peoples Service Drug Store v. Somerville-1932,* a pharmacist filled a prescription for 1/4 grain strychnine capsules that resulted in injury. The prescription was filled properly according to the physician's order. The issue was whether a pharmacist's failure to consult a physician regarding the unusual dosage of the drug was a direct cause of the patient's injuries. The court ruled against the pharmacist stating that pharmacists had the duty to contradict the physician only when medication orders were obviously fatal, and to simply make an inquiry of the physician when an order appeared to be non-life-threatening but unusual.[1]

Much later, the 1986 landmark case of *Riff v. Morgan Pharmacy* began to open the floodgates for litigation against pharmacists. The facts of the case are that the plaintiff, Patricia Riff, experienced severe migraine headaches. She went to her physician and received a prescription for Cafergot Suppositories, a potent vasopressor. She brought the prescription to the pharmacy which was then filled with the following directions: "Insert one suppository rectally every four hours for headache." No other instructions or warnings were given and no refills were authorized. After using some four suppositories, the headache subsided.

A few months later, Mrs. Riff experienced another headache and used up the remainder of her prescription. Feeling no relief, she refilled the prescription and used some 15 to 17 suppositories over a 4-day period. These events were again repeated a short time later except this time she began to experience discomfort in her foot and leg. Upon visiting the hospital, it was determined that the cause of the discomfort was Cafergot overdose and that there was a possibility that she could die, or at the very least, lose her leg through a required amputation. The Riffs brought suit against the pharmacist for not warning the plaintiff that the maximum dosage for Cafergot Suppositories was not more than five suppositories per week and for illegally filling the prescription without authorization. The jury returned a verdict that the pharmacist was 65% at fault. The court stated: "Expert testimony established that the 'reasonable pharmacist' has an affirmative duty to read the prescription and to be aware of patent inadequacies in the instructions as to the maximum safe dosage of known toxic drugs and medicines. Morgan Pharmacy failed in that duty."[2]

As demonstrated in *Riff*, pharmacists can now be held to a far higher level of practice accountability than they were in *Peoples*. If clinical and advocacy models of pharmacy practice are shaping the pharmacist's standard and duty to care, what does the law require? Simply, a pharmacist is "required to use that degree of care which a reasonable and prudent person would use under similar circumstances," and "a pharmacist is bound to exercise the skill generally possessed by well-educated pharmacists who are considered competent in their profession, rather than the highest skill and learning, which can only be obtained by a few men and women of rare genius, endowments or opportunities."[3]

As a practical matter, pharmacists must practice error free. The slightest mistake can result in an injury. Therefore, when an injury can be avoided through some action yet the action is not taken, the duty of care has been breached. This discussion suggests that smart and proper thinking applies to the courts' interpretation of when pharmacists are liable. If the standard by which a pharmacist will be judged is to do something such as using a "smart rule strategy," and one decides not do that something, that pharmacist is liable.

To further illustrate this distinction, in the 1985 case of *Ingram v. Hook's Drugs, Inc.*, the court ruled that if pharmacists included all of the warnings listed for each prescription medication as described in the United States

Pharmacopeia Dispensing Information* on a prescription container, "Such voluminous warnings would only confuse that normal customer and be of dubious value. The matter is better handled by the treating physician."[4]

A 1991 appellate decision of the Illinois case of *Frye v. Medicare-Glazer Corporation*[5] regarding a patient who was prescribed the drug Fiorinal for pain offers additional insights on these issues.** The pharmacist who filled the prescription attached a warning label to the container which indicated that the drug had a tendency to cause drowsiness. The patient then drank a quantity of alcohol and died. The estate filed a complaint against the pharmacist alleging that although there was no duty to warn the decedent of the dangerous effects of the drug, once she undertook the duty to warn and did so negligently (the estate contends that the warning was incomplete in that the effects with alcohol were not included along with drowsiness), she was responsible for the death of Mr. Frye. The appellate court overturned the lower court ruling and stated that the plaintiff may maintain an action against the pharmacist who voluntarily assumes a duty to warn of a drug's adverse reactions, but does so in an incomplete manner. The court's reasoning was that, "a consumer who receives a warning from a pharmacist is entitled to rely upon the accuracy and completeness of that warning. A consumer who receives no warning from the pharmacist must consult his physician to obtain additional information."[5] The Illinois Supreme Court later heard this case and overturned the appellate court's decision. "The majority opinion found that the only responsibility that the pharmacist assumed was to warn Frye about drowsiness, which she did without negligence, and "The supreme court judges rejected the appellate courts ruling, reasoning that it would have a chilling effect on patient counseling. If pharmacists who warn of some side effects could be held liable for not disclosing all the side effects of a drug, the justices opined that pharmacists, 'would refrain from placing any warning labels on containers,' thus depriving all consumers of all warnings."[6]

The judges further stated, "In our opinion, consumers should primarily look to their prescribing physician to convey the appropriate warnings regarding drugs, and it is the prescribing physician's duty to convey these warnings to patients."[6] Thus, in *Frye*, the courts have taken the seemingly traditional philosophy that the physician has the duty and not the pharmacist.

Lawsuits heard by the courts in the 1970s and 1980s regarding a pharmacist's duty to warn were predominantly decided on the issue of whether a pharmacist had the duty or not. Cases such as *Riff v. Morgan Pharmacy*[2] in which pharmacists were held liable for failing to warn patients against the more dangerous effects of prescribed drugs are widely discussed by pharmacy's professional press. The majority of cases results in decisions that hold

---

* The United States Pharmacopeia Dispensing Information is the accepted official compendia for medication standards, prescribing and patient information. In Massachusetts, it is required.
** Fiorinal is a combination product containing butabarbital and aspirin manufactured by Sandoz Pharmaceuticals. Due to its addictive potential, Fiorinal is a federally controlled substance listed in Schedule III. It is used in the treatment of migraine headache.

pharmacists to be outside the loop of the physician–patient relationship, and in many of those cases where the pharmacist is held to be liable, it was only because the pharmacist gratuitously undertook to provide a warning but did so incorrectly. More simply stated, the courts really do not understand what it is that pharmacists can actually do, hence, cannot hold the profession liable if it fails to do something.[7]

The expectation was that OBRA '90 would fundamentally change all of this. The legislation spelled out in a reasonably concise format what is expected of a pharmacist within the context of the healthcare system. The courts had something in print, in the law, from which to evaluate whether a pharmacist did something properly or not. The idea that pharmacists can do something is not new. Past studies from the Office of the U.S. Inspector General reported that pharmacists as professionals could impact the cost and quality of healthcare in a very positive way, yet they also found that pharmacists failed to do so.[8] The profession strongly responded that we were treated unfairly and that we do the things, such as counseling patients, that the government alleged we did not.

In practice, OBRA's requirements still place a heavy burden on the practicing pharmacist. There are few other, if any, practitioners in the health-care field who interact daily with the large number of patients that community pharmacists do. While counseling a patient about proper medication use will improve drug therapy outcomes and globally be more cost effective than poor or noncompliance, such counseling will render the pharmacist's time less efficient when measured by prescription volume. This may be of concern to some in light of OBRA's nonreimbursement for cognitive services and predicted savings in healthcare as a result of those services. These issues, however, are not legally sufficient as the basis for a pharmacist's noncompliance with OBRA. Indeed, the courts and regulatory bodies are bound to uphold laws enacted by the legislature unless there is some basis in law not to do so.

Issues

The expanded role for pharmacy as envisioned by OBRA '90 included patient care services that make the pharmacist a more significant player in healthcare delivery. Any time someone is directed to perform more responsibilities, however, such as drug use review and patient counseling, there is an increased risk of making an error for which that person could be held legally liable. Even in the year 2002, pharmacists appear to be aware of, rather than fearful of, the legal implications of their expanding function in the increasingly integrated system of healthcare delivery.[9]

A few court cases in recent years have held pharmacists liable under the legal concept of "negligence," and in these cases, the conduct of the pharmacist has been found to be sufficiently wanting as judged by relevant professional standards on pharmaceutical care, resulting in the payment of monetary damages to the plaintiff by the pharmacist defendant. In each of these legal battles, the plaintiff was required to prove in court, through the use of expert witnesses and other evidence, that the conduct in question was in fact negligent according to legally proven standards of "reasonable" pharmaceutical care. Generally, courts have avoided imposing duties on the practice of pharmacy that were not legislatively mandated; to do so would be to state public policy which is the province of a state legislature.[10]

The directives contained in OBRA '90 and in the subsequent laws and regulations passed by the states codify or provide for specific laws and regulations that specify the duties of pharmacists in the treatment of patients who receive prescriptions. This means that the failure to comply with these duties will automatically be considered negligence without the necessity of the plaintiff proving through evidence that there was a duty. For example, in Massachusetts, the law specifies that if the offer to counsel is accepted, the pharmacists shall if appropriate discuss with patients the proper storage of prescribed medications.[11] As a result, no time will be spent at trial presenting evidence to prove or disprove whether or not a pharmacist actually had a duty, or a legal obligation, to discuss medication storage because the law states plainly and clearly that he or she does. This legal concept is referred to as "negligence per se." As before, the plaintiff, however, will still have to show that he or she was harmed, and that this harm was actually caused by the negligent conduct found. However, one very important note of caution needs to be remembered. The fact that a violation of a statute or regulation is considered "negligence per se," does not mean that simple conformance with that statute or regulation signifies that a pharmacist has acted "reasonably" in the legal sense. What is reasonable conduct depends upon the circumstances of each individual situation, and it is certainly conceivable that a pharmacist could be found negligent for failure to take precautions beyond the bare minimum implied by statutory compliance.

It should be noted that the original directives of OBRA '90 apply only to Medicaid patients. This point has become moot because most state legislatures or boards of registration in pharmacy have decided to create laws or promulgate regulations to make the OBRA '90 standards applicable to all patients. As early as 1992, the Massachusetts legislature changed its laws to include all patients with new prescriptions. In 1998, the Massachusetts Board promulgated its own regulations, further defining the Chapter 94c mandates of maintaining patient records, conducting prospective drug utilization review, and patient counseling.[12]

With the maturation of pharmacy practice into an even greater patient care-oriented profession, professional standards will be fluid and evolving, so mere technical compliance with these new mandates may not be legally or professionally adequate or reasonable. It is important for pharmacists — as for all healthcare professionals — to realize that the law is not a natural science. The law is an ever-mutating construct, always trying to graft the notion of "fairness" or "justice" onto new developments in technology, knowledge, or human activity.

The best approach for pharmacists concerned about the legal implications of their legislated responsibilities then is to understand compliance with them from the patient's point of view. What is reasonable from the viewpoint of the patient with regard to drug use review or patient counseling? It may be helpful to consider the intent behind the standards imposed. Drug Use Review (DUR) provisions appear to be an effort to amplify the communication between patients, physicians, and pharmacists to enhance patient outcomes, such as compliance with prescribed medication regimes, which in turn should boost the cost effectiveness of drug therapy.

Prospective drug review

For a pharmacist's patient-counseling activity to be meaningful, counseling must be performed within the context of patient-specific information. Traditionally, prior to filling a prescription the pharmacist would perform a prospective review of the prescription to establish the prescription's correctness (dosage, frequency, and other requirements) and authenticity. In such a review, the pharmacist could be held negligent if the pharmacist breached the duty of ordinary care and diligence.[13] Unless the patient was asked to or voluntarily provided specific personal information for use by the pharmacist (such as allergies, concurrent medication use, or other information) no other review for the patient's benefit was usually performed; the pharmacist acted on the basis that any and all other aspects of prescription drug therapy were addressed by the prescriber. However, once the pharmacist has specific patient information, the pharmacist must utilize that information and provide correct advice.[14]

Under OBRA, however, the specific requirement of a prospective drug review can be accomplished only by collecting and assessing patient-specific information prior to filling the prescription. This requirement necessitates solicitation of patient-specific information before filling or delivering the prescription to the patient or patient's caregiver. If a problem such as therapeutic duplication, drug-disease contraindication, adverse drug–drug interaction, etc. is identified by the pharmacist[15] as a result of the review, an active pharmacist intervention with the prescriber for the patient's benefit should occur.[16]

Really ... what's it all mean?

The counseling laws and regulations as now defined under present law and regulation raise some interesting issues. The question still lingers in the minds of many pharmacists whether we really have to counsel or have to offer to counsel. The simple answer is that we are only required to *offer* counseling. This is clear in both our laws and regulations. However, we are expected by the public and, to a great degree by professional standards, to actually conduct counseling. The downside to not counseling is that in the event of any problem experienced by a patient, pharmacists who legally choose not to counsel will face the somewhat daunting burden of defending and justifying that decision. So, one assumes that it is just easier to counsel to some degree and deal with the supposed lesser issue of "counseling lite."

One difficult aspect of OBRA is the requirement to warn about common severe adverse or side effects.[17] While pharmacy practitioners may accept specific directions as to the extent or quantity of warning that must be provided for compliance with this requirement, it may be troubling to some because it may not be adequate to preclude a negligence suit for not warning sufficiently.[10] It is usually not possible to state with absolute certainty which severe side or adverse effect(s) will occur in a particular patient each time that person's prescription is filled or refilled. Additionally, side effects and/or adverse effects are commonly the result of a patient taking or using the prescribed drug. Under OBRA, the pharmacist must, however, provide information about which side effects and adverse effects will occur before and/or while the patient takes or uses the drug. Some are concerned that it will be of little comfort to a patient counseled about, for example, three adverse effects of a drug when the patient is seriously harmed by the drug's fourth adverse effect.

Conclusion

As the pharmacy profession grapples with the implications of the edicts of OBRA '90, those pharmacists who base their professional activities on their ability to empathize with the needs of their patients should have little or no trouble being in legal compliance. This point is an important one. One of the more common pharmaceutical refrains is, "My patients never ask me anything." From the patient's perspective, however, most pharmacies are hardly designed to be conducive to private inquiries or discussions about matters that are highly personal or intimate.

It seems likely that the new obligations of OBRA '90 will cause the redesign of the pharmacy environment to accommodate the goals, and there are studies under way to determine the best ways to achieve this. From a practical standpoint, those pharmacists who practice "OBRA pharmacy" in the fulfillment of their newly minted legal and professional obligations should have little to worry about from a liability perspective. OBRA '90, in fact, does little more than spell out the manner by which pharmacists should be complying with the Code of Ethics of the American Pharmaceutical Association, which requires pharmacists to hold the health and safety of their patients to be their main consideration and to respect the confidential and personal nature of patient drug profiles. It would even seem fair to predict that enthusiastic or aggressive compliance with the dictates of OBRA '90 will lead to a possible reduction in the risk of legal liabilities for pharmacists, despite the newly codified imposition of affirmative pharmaceutical obligations.

Bibliography

1. *Peoples Service Drug Stores v. Somerville*, 158 A. 12 (Md. 1932).
2. *Riff v. Morgan*, 508 A.2d 1247 (Pa. Super. 1986).
3. *Hoar v. Rasmussen*, 282 N.W. 652 (Wis. 1938).
4. *Ingram v. Hook's Drugs, Inc.*, 476 N.E. 2nd 881 (Ind. Ct. App. 1985).
5. *Frye v. Medicare-Glazer Corporation*, No. 5-90-0559, Ill. App. Ct. 5th Dist. October 8, 1991.
6. R.Ph.'s duty to warn short-circuited for now, *Drug Topics*, November 23, 1992, 14.
7. Brushwood, D., *Pharmacy Law Annual 1988*, 4.
8. Anon., The Clinical Role of the Community Pharmacist, U.S. Department of Health and Human Services, Office of the Inspector General, Nov. 1990.
9. Pisano, D., A study exploring regulatory coping behaviors in community practice, Presented Papers Session for the American Society of Pharmacy Law, American Pharmaceutical Association, 145th Annual Meeting, Miami, FL, March 1998 (Podium).
10. *McKee v. American Home Products*, 782 P. 2nd 1045 (Wash. Sup. Ct. Nov. 30, 1989).
11. Chapter 94c, Sec. 21a, (6).
12. 247CMR9.07, et seq.
13. *Ferguson v. Williams*, 374 S.E. 2nd 438 (N.C. App. 1988).
14. *Frye v. Medicare-Glaser Corp.*, 579 N.E. 2d 1255, Ill. App. Ct. 5th Dist. Oct. 8, 1991 in Brushwood, D., Pharmacy Law Annual 1998.
15. 57 Fed. Reg. No.112, 49409, Nov. 2, 1992.
16. *Hendricks v. Charity Hospital of New Orleans*, 519 So. 2nd, 163 (La. App. 4 Cir. 1987).
17. 57 Fed. Regis. No. 212, 49410, Nov. 2, 1992.

chapter six

Pharmaceutical care: Our legal and professional strategic plan

Healthcare is a people-helping-people profession. All members of the health-care team are well aware of the responsibilities to do no harm and promote healing and comfort. Since the early 1990s, pharmacists, pharmacy students, and to an increasing degree, pharmacy technicians are being asked to continue to assert this role in the care and treatment of patients. We in the profession have dubbed this activity "pharmaceutical care." Pharmaceutical care is the basic concept of care by the pharmacist through the use of medications and specialized knowledge that will increase the quality of life from the patient's perspective. The purpose of this chapter is to discuss many, though not all, of the basic elements of pharmaceutical care, the reasons for its importance in the current state of pharmacy practice, its risk management properties, and the strategic elements for practice in the 21st century.

The Pew Commission reports and the changing landscape of healthcare

In 1995, the Pew Commission published a number of reports that described the current and future status of U.S. healthcare. The third report of the series entitled "Critical Challenges: Revitalizing the Health Professions for the Twenty-First Century" was published in November 1995.[1] It was intended to be a guide for those healthcare professionals and their organizations who intended to survive the transformation dynamics of the current healthcare system and thrive in the emerging healthcare culture. This report was particularly important to practitioners because it made suggestions about what was needed in healthcare and, therefore, opened the door to pharmaceutical care.

The report suggested that, in general, American society needed to address several key issues such as the ways in which the work of health professionals is organized; the ways in which health professionals are regulated; the size, education, and organization of the health workforce; and the skills that professionals bring to the workplace. The report suggested that the current healthcare system was inefficient and expensive. Many of the functions of health professionals and their agencies are redundant, overlapping, territorial, and slow. Also, the regulation of healthcare uses an older, autocratic model where regulatory agencies may be more punitive than introspective, and reactive rather than innovative. In addition, the report stressed the need to change the educational process to train a more multidimensional health professional who is able to practice more globally in response to healthcare need rather than the current, somewhat narrow, professional model. Clearly, the report suggested that for it to survive, the U.S. healthcare system needed to deconstruct itself, and tear down its rules, professional boundaries, and inefficient practices and accounting to reinvent itself into a more efficient, accessible system.

Strong words indeed! The report predicted closure of 50% of hospitals and loss of 60% of beds due to a massive expansion of primary care in ambulatory and community settings. Much of this may have come to pass as the closure of smaller community hospitals has become a reality, especially for those unaffiliated with larger hospitals and as a patient's length of stay for more routine procedures has given way to day surgery and outpatient care. In addition, the report suggested that, in the future, there may be a large surplus of healthcare professionals. For example, the report posits that there may be 100,000–150,000 too many physicians due to less demand for specialists, 200,000–300,000 excess nurses as hospitals close, and some 40,000 more pharmacists than needed as dispensing is automated or centralized. Also, a fundamental alteration may be needed in the ways health profession schools educate their students by consolidating many of the traditional health professions into a single multi-skilled profession as health systems are redesigned, i.e., a nurse practitioner/physician assistant model where diagnosing, prescribing, etc. may be conducted in a more cost-efficient fashion.

For example, the report recommended that pharmacy:

> Reduce the number of pharmacy schools by 20 to 25% by the year 2005!!
> Maintain only those pharmacy schools located in regions of the country where there is need
> Focus professional training more on issues of clinical pharmacy, systems management, and work with other health providers

Of note, the report suggested that a reduction in pharmacy schools had merit. However, it is interesting to see that in the early 2000s, there continues to be keen interest in opening additional pharmacy schools all over the country. However, the more germane aspect of their recommendations lay in the suggested focus of our professional training. As discussed in Chapter

1, The Evolution of Pharmacy Practice, our professional curricula have evolved from the technical to the clinical and practice management modes. This recommendation created the overwhelming conditions that foster pharmaceutical care and the pharmaceutical care model as the structure of our professional strategic plan.

Pharmaceutical care and the pharmaceutical care model

Pharmaceutical care first hit the pharmacy scene in 1990. It was term coined by Drs. C. Douglas Hepler and Linda Strand,[2] in their article, "Opportunities and Responsibilities in Pharmaceutical Care" published in the *American Journal of Health Systems Pharmacy*. In this article, pharmaceutical care was defined as "the responsible provision of drug therapy for the purpose of achieving definite outcomes that improve the patient's overall quality of life." This is the defining purpose of pharmacy practice!

What is quality of life? It certainly means different things to different people. From a patient's perspective, quality of life may mean being able to dress one's self or take a pleasant stroll with a spouse, family, or friends, or simply, having the proper medication to alleviate painful or otherwise troubling symptoms of medications used to treat an illness. Quality of life may certainly be decided by the effectiveness of the pharmacist in his or her role as patient advocate. The effectiveness can be measured in terms of outcomes or the measurable result of one's efforts on behalf of the patient.[3]

In pharmacy, the term "outcomes" has virtually become a household word. Outcomes are defined as cure of disease, elimination or reduction of symptomatology, arresting or slowing of disease, or prevention of disease or symptomatology. Not as lofty as they may seem. For example, HIV/AIDS has become a chronic rather than an acute disease through the use of multi-drug "cocktails," and conditions such arthritis, asthma, diabetes, and osteoporosis have become somewhat easier for patients to cope with due to current therapeutic modalities. All require medication and that the pharmacist "do something" such as counseling or drug use review.

The issue of "doing something" leads us to the next step, the "Pharmaceutical Care Model." The pharmaceutical care model empowers pharmacists to encourage patients to assume responsibility for drug therapy within the framework of their own lifestyle, values, and environmental factors. This is accomplished by identifying, resolving, and/or preventing potential and actual drug-related problems. It requires an expanded role and expanded duty for the pharmacy professional! The pharmaceutical care model dictates that pharmacists act on behalf of and in the best interest of the patient from the patient's perspective. For example, if patients have arthritic hands and require half-tablets of their medications and cannot break them themselves, the pharmaceutical care model would dictate this simple action. In another example, a patient's busy caregiver would be well served by the pharmacist who takes the time to develop a clear and concise medication administration plan that helps the caregiver properly administer medication on time.

Pharmaceutical care may be condensed into the following five simple steps or principles.[4]

1. Know your patient
2. Keep good records
3. Develop a plan
4. Empower the patient
5. Follow up

Principle 1: Know your patient

A professional relationship must be established and maintained. It is incumbent upon a pharmacist to take the time and effort to know each and every patient to the fullest extent possible. In many community and long-term care practices, pharmacists may be on a first name basis with a majority of their patients. Over time, this familiarity will foster mutual trust and respect, a pharmacist–patient relationship. This relationship sets the stage for in-depth interview and discussion with a patient about his or her medications and concerns. It also gives the pharmacist an idea of who the patient is on a cultural and personal level. For example, many elderly patients may feel uncomfortable discussing their medical problems with anyone including their physicians. They may make statements such as, "we didn't discuss those things in my day." Knowing this may aid the pharmacist in developing an alternative means of acquiring and sharing information sensitive to the patient.

Principle 2: Keep good records

Patient-specific medical information must be collected, organized, recorded, maintained, and evaluated. At this point in the evolution of pharmacy practice, record keeping and the associated technology used to maintain it are fairly standard practices. The issue arises in evaluating data. Clearly, the effort by many state boards of pharmacy to require a prospective drug use review by pharmacists prior to dispensing new prescriptions and subsequent counseling about them has fostered a more prevalent data evaluation, or patient profile review.

Principle 3: Develop a plan

A drug therapy plan must be developed and mutually agreed upon with the patient. The pharmaceutical care model empowers the pharmacist to encourage patients to assume responsibility for drug therapy within the framework of their own life styles, values, and environmental factors. This requires a clear and concise plan that is acceptable to the patient and achieves the goals or outcomes as dictated by their therapy or their decisions about therapy. Simple verbal plans may be better than none at all and may suffice for some patients on simple maintenance therapy. Taking medications before meals or after them or at bedtime or earlier may appear mundane to many pharmacy practitioners, but is of tantamount importance to the patient who experiences nausea, nocturnal bladder urges, or drowsiness. Therefore, more may need to be considered than is apparent when developing even a simple medication plan.

Principle 4: Empower the patient

The pharmacist assures that the patient has the supplies, information, and knowledge necessary to carry out the drug therapy plan. While developing a plan is difficult enough, a pharmacist must also be aware that the patient may need some degree of education or training to successfully carry out the agreed-upon plan. Does the patient understand how to use his or her inhaler, aerochamber, glucose monitoring kit, blood pressure cuff, stethoscope, suppository, cream, ointment, etc.? Does the patient understand how his or her medical condition differs from the neighbors? Can he repeat your instructions back to you? Is he comfortable with all that was discussed and agreed to in the plan? If the answer is "yes," the patient may be sufficiently empowered to "assume responsibility for their drug therapy within the framework of their own life style, values, and environmental factors."

Principle 5: Follow up

The pharmacist reviews, monitors, and modifies the therapeutic plan as necessary and appropriate, in concert with the patient and health team. After achieving some success with Principles 1 through 4, the difficult step is yet to come. It deals with the issues associated with compliance. Compliance is not only the patient's concern in the pharmaceutical care model, it reaches out to the profession as well. The diagnosis of a medical condition and the prescription of a medication used to treat it are not of a single dimension. More likely, the review and monitoring of a patient's medication plan may resemble an algorithm with a number of "if x, then y" pathways with which to contend and make decisions about. Who better than the pharmacist to check in with a patient at the time of refill or when she enters the pharmacy for reasons other than prescription filling to find out how her treatment is going. Better yet, pharmacy software systems are being developed and used to prompt the pharmacist when a patient diverts from a prior agreed-upon medication plan or automatically e-mails or calls the patient when a refill is due. However, as convenient as this technology may be, pharmaceutical care is better served when the pharmacist calls the patient directly some number of days after therapy has been initiated. This principle may still require the most work!!!!

Therefore, at present, four of the five Principles of Pharmaceutical Care are more or less accomplished through common daily practice modalities at each and every site. However, to continue to use pharmaceutical care as our professional strategic plan, the fifth principle will require continued attention as the profession progresses. One must remember, pharmaceutical care is a necessary element of healthcare that provides for the direct benefit of the patient, holding the pharmacist directly responsible for the patient's care.

Rudimentary pharmaceutical care equals counseling!!!!

In the famous words of Sherlock Holmes, "It's elementary my dear Watson," patient counseling is one of the most rudimentary forms of pharmaceutical care. Counseling regulations have been established by boards of pharmacy in many states for a number of reasons including the enhancement of the patient health and welfare by requiring pharmacists to offer counseling, promoting optimum therapeutic outcomes, avoiding patient injury, and reducing medication errors. It is in these regulations that one may begin to view pharmaceutical care as a risk management strategy used to prevent and/or protect the pharmacy practitioner against lawsuits or other liabilities.

Many states have counseling regulations that require pharmacists to *do* something, such as the requirement to keep a confidential patient record (Principle #2), conduct a prospective drug use review before each new prescription is dispensed or delivered to a patient to promote therapeutic appropriateness (Principles #2 and #3), and take appropriate action which may include consultation with the prescriber or patient upon the identification of inappropriate therapeutics to ensure proper patient care (Principle #5).

In addition, federal OBRA '90 regulations as well the laws and regulations of many states require an "offer to counsel" by a pharmacist or designee who shall offer the services of the pharmacist to discuss issues that in the pharmacist's professional judgment are deemed to be significant for the health and safety of the patient. The pharmacist's professional judgment refers to decisions that the pharmacist is expected to make based on knowledge of the patient and the patient's medical situation (Principle #1). It should also be mentioned that in the offer of the services of the pharmacist, there is an underlying assumption that those services are cognitive and require a higher-level specialized expertise that may only be delivered by the pharmacist. The offer to counsel is made to the patient or to the person acting on behalf of the patient (as permitted by local law or regulation) when confidentiality can be maintained, either by face-to-face communication or by telephone, or a written offer may be provided if the prescription is not picked up by the patient or not made by telephone. A pharmacist may provide such information which, in the pharmacist's professional judgment, is necessary for the patient to understand the proper use of the prescription (Principles #1, #4, and #5).

Pharmaceutical care and risk management

Risk management is loosely defined as a series or a system of techniques used to minimize negative outcomes from common activities. It is designed to reduce the incidence of administrative, cognitive, clinical, and technical errors. In community practice, risk management must include OBRA '90!!! However, pharmacy risk management is not risk elimination and, in health-care, some risk is necessary to benefit patients. For example, the old adage that "the cure is worse than the disease" may hold true for many patients. Therefore, some medications may be the therapy of choice even though they can cause unwanted side effects or adverse reactions. Many of these unwanted side effects or adverse reactions are known and minimized successfully with some careful forethought.

However, the value of pharmaceutical care is that it promotes effective risk management by encompassing a system that reduces the incidence of preventable error and lessens the consequences of error that cannot be prevented. The system?

1. Know your patient
2. Keep good records
3. Develop a plan
4. Empower the patient
5. Follow up

Interestingly, the courts are beginning to understand that pharmacists are playing a significant role in the care of patients. Here are some examples.

In the case of *Griffin v. Phar-Mor, Inc.,* [9] however, the issue was whether a pharmacy that makes a dispensing error is guilty of fraud and misrepresentation so as to extend the statute of limitations; the significance of this lies in the statements by the court. In this case the drug Maxzide was dispensed for the drug Micronase. The patient took the wrong drug unknowingly and became ill. When she called the pharmacy, she was informed of the error and decided to sue. The court agreed that the patient was wronged because the pharmacy did not inform her of the error. The court stated, "The relationship between a pharmacist and the client is one in which the client puts extreme trust in the pharmacist." Further, "Pharmacists possess important specialized knowledge that is possessed by few, if any nonpharmacists, and it is this specialized knowledge that puts patients in the position of having to put complete trust and confidence in the pharmacists skill." If this does not represent an argument for pharmaceutical care, maybe the next case will be more convincing.

In the case of *Hooks SuperX, Inc. v. McLaughlin*, the issue was, "Whether a pharmacist has a duty to cease refilling prescriptions for a patient who is receiving controlled substances (CSs) at an unreasonably faster rate than the rate prescribed without receiving explicit directions of the physician."[10] In this case, a patient had a history of back injury and had been using large quantities of propoxyphene for a long period of time. The treating physician, realizing that the patient was overusing the drug, refused to issue further prescriptions to him. The patient became despondent and attempted suicide. Later he sued the pharmacist for filling the prescriptions that the pharmacist should have known would injure his health (a breach of a duty to care).

Professors David Brushwood and Richard Abood in their book *Pharmacy Practice and the Law*[11] suggest that this case examines a pharmacist's expanded duty to conduct pharmaceutical care based on three factors: relationship, foreseeability, and public policy. The court recognized that there is a direct pharmacist–patient relationship which is sufficiently close to justify imposing a duty (to intervene), and that a pharmacist's knowledge of medications and the patient makes the probability of harm to the patient foreseeable, and that good public policy supports this duty by preventing intentional/unintentional drug use, not jeopardizing the physician–patient relationship, and avoiding unnecessary health costs. All convincing and powerful arguments that pharmaceutical care is necessary in the strategic and legal aspects of pharmacy practice.

The strategic plan

The strategic plan for pharmaceutical care should encompass the five main goals listed under *Pharmaceutical care and risk management*. Each has subcomponents and must be evaluated or reevaluated as professional of healthcare changes. Recommendations on the implementation of a pharmaceutical care strategic plan will center on pharmacists, pharmacy schools, and pharmacy boards.

Pharmacists

Pharmacists need to identify appropriate indicators and oversight mechanisms to ensure that professional behavior leads to measurable patient outcomes.

More simply, how do we measure our performance? Some tools that could be used include

- Comprehensive drug therapy management
  The primary goal of drug therapy management is to improve patient outcomes in a cost-effective manner through a collaborative process of selecting appropriate drug therapies, educating patients, monitoring patients, and continually assessing outcomes of therapy.
- Performance measurement
  Performance measurement requires a wide array of experts who have the experience and knowledge to develop benchmarks (points of reference) and sentinel event indicators (indicators that require immediate investigation) as quantitative indicators, such as the number of patients returning for refills within a given month, or some number of prescription filling errors considered as excessive over a predetermined period of time.

Peer review

Peer review mechanisms need to be formed from the profession's members, its customers, and other stakeholders. It must be created to expediently decide on the appropriateness of behavior, accountability for controlling costs, enhancing patient and consumer satisfaction, and improving health-care outcomes. This may be accomplished through credentialing.

Credentialing

Credentialing is the process by which an organization or institution obtains, verifies, and assesses a pharmacist's qualifications to provide patient care services. Credentialing indicates to society that a pharmacist is qualified to practice at an advanced level. Why? Pharmacists and the profession are faced with increasing complexity in healthcare, a push toward expanded roles, possible future requirements for professional competency, and the prospect of reimbursement for cognitive services.

There are many types of credentialing that may be of interest to pharmacists. These include academic postgraduate education (i.e., nontraditional Pharm.D., Master's degree programs), residencies (institutional or community), clinical fellowships, traineeships that are short and intensive, and topic-specific courses and certificate programs that are "shorter than a degree, longer than training" and generally require ongoing competency. Some examples of certifying agencies for pharmacists include the Board of Pharmaceutical Specialties (BPS) of the American Pharmaceutical Association (which certifies for nuclear pharmacy, nutrition support, oncology, pharmacotherapy, psychiatric pharmacy), and the Commission for Certification in Geriatric Pharmacy (CCGP) of the American Society of Consultant Pharmacists. In addition, the National Institute for Standards in Pharmacist Credentialing (NISPC) was founded jointly by the American Pharmaceutical Association (APhA), the National Association of Boards of Pharmacy (NABP), the National Association of Chain Drug Stores (NACDS), and the National Community Pharmacists Association (NCPA). Its purpose is to promote the value of and encourage the adoption of the NABP disease-specific examinations as the consistent and objective means of documenting the ability of pharmacists to provide disease state management (DSM) services. These certifications include anticoagulation, asthma, diabetes, and dyslipidemia.

Pharmacy schools

Pharmacy's academic institutions must continue to reconfigure their educational programs to establish better alliances with stakeholders of pharmaceutical care.

Pharmacy schools must continue to reinforce the basics of clinical practice, pharmacy business administration, and health systems management within the curricular designs. In addition, pharmacy schools are changing and reevaluating their experiential training to be more broad based including hospital, general medicine, managed care, and community pharmacy.

Pharmacy boards

Pharmacy's regulatory bodies are continuing to standardize practice requirements to facilitate professional competence and induce flexibility in existing licensing laws through the minimization of public regulation.

Many pharmacy boards are working toward a vision of Uniform Practice Standards and Policies that will help standardize regulations between states through continuing competency initiatives, i.e., continuous quality improvement (CQI) to assess and improve the level of pharmacy practice of their licensees, and regulatory flexibility that permits pharmacists and pharmacies to make a case for their actions based on the best interest of the patients they serve.

Conclusion

Pharmaceutical care is the hallmark of the profession. It explains what it is that a practitioner of pharmacy can do to promote the health of patients. It requires personal involvement by all members of the profession, some additional training, and much in the way of public relations. It has all of the elements for strategic planning, gives direction, has vision, and is attainable. As we have seen, the courts are beginning to understand that pharmaceutical care has impact on the general public and this is good! There has probably never been so much opportunity for the pharmacy practitioner, colleges, and boards of registration to have as much impact as there is today.

Bibliography

1. Pew Health Professions Commission, *Critical Challenges: Revitalizing the Health Professions for the Twenty-First Century*, USCF Center for the Health Professions, San Francisco, CA, 1995.
2. Hepler, C.D. and Strand, L., Opportunities and responsibilities in pharmaceutical care, *American Journal of Health Systems Pharmacy*, 47:533-43, 1990.
3. McDowell, I. and Newell, C., *Measuring Health: A Guide to Rating Scales and Questionnaires*, Oxford University Press, New York, 1987, p. 204.
4. Rovers, J. et al., *A Practical Guide to Pharmaceutical Care*, 1st ed., American Pharmaceutical Association, 1998.
5. *Peoples Service Drug Stores v. Somerville*, 158 A. 12 (Md.1932).
6. *Hoar v. Rasmussen*, 282 N.W. 652 (Wis. 1938).
7. *Frye v. Medicare-Glazer Corporation*, No. 5-90-0559, Ill. App. Ct. 5th Dist. October 8, 1991.
8. R.Ph.'s duty to warn short-circuited for now, *Drug Topics*, November 23, 1992, p. 14.
9. *Griffin v. Phar-Mor, Inc.*, 790 F. Supp. 1115 (S.D. Ala. 1992).

10. *Hooks SuperX, Inc. v. McLaughlin,* 642 N.E. 2nd 514 (Ind. 1994).
11. Abood, R. and Brushwood, D., *Pharmacy Practice and the Law,* 3rd ed., Aspen Publishing, Gaithersburg, MD, 2001, pp. 330–331.

part two

Case studies in pharmacy law

chapter seven

Case studies

Controlled Substances Act

Case #1

Dr. Williams Peters calls you at your community pharmacy and asks you to fill a prescription for a controlled substance in Schedule II in an emergency supply for John Smith, a mounted police officer and a long-time patron of your pharmacy. You inquire as to the nature of the emergency and the prescriber indicates that Officer Smith has a hairline fracture in his right ankle that he incurred while dismounting his police horse.

The physician prescribes:

Oxycodone with acetaminophen tablets   #30
Sig: Take one tablet every six hours as needed for pain.
No Refills   DEA# AP1357938

You request a hard-copy, written prescription to be mailed to you. Instead, Dr. Peters faxes the prescription to your pharmacy. However, before you have the opportunity to have the prescription delivered, the patient painfully walks into your pharmacy and requests the prescription. You fill and dispense the prescription.

Questions
1. Which of the following factors is/are false regarding the dispensing of an emergency supply of CIIs without a prescription?
   a. The patient needs the drug right away.
   b. The physician cannot get a written prescription to the patient or pharmacy.
   c. A Schedule III controlled substance will not alleviate the pain.
   d. The physician has 72 hours to mail a hard copy to the patient.
   e. The physician has 7 days to mail a hard copy to the pharmacist.
   f. Answers a, b, and c

g. Answers a, b, c, and e
h. Answers a, b, c, and d
i. Answer d
j. Answer e

2. Which of the following DEA numbers is correct for William Peters, M.D.?
   a. AP 1357938
   b. RP 1221390
   c. AP 1221388
   d. AP 3798611
   e. AW 1256734

3. If this prescriber telephoned an emergency prescription order for a CIV such as propoxyphene (rather than a CII) into the pharmacy, how long would that prescriber have to send or mail a hard-copy prescription to the pharmacy to comply with the federal CSA?
   a. 72 hours
   b. 48 hours
   c. 7 days
   d. 5 days
   e. None required under federal law

4. Which of the following faxed prescriptions may be kept as an original prescription (in place of a handwritten hard copy) for CII drugs?
   a. Prescriptions for solid, oral dosage forms for ambulatory patients living at home and who are chronically ill.
   b. Prescriptions for intravenous dosage forms for patients with terminal illness.
   c. Prescriptions for solid, oral dosage forms for patients in long-term care facilities.
   d. Answers a and b may be kept as original prescriptions.
   e. Answers b and c may be kept as original prescriptions.

5. With regard to the presented case and according to federal laws and regulations, the pharmacist filling this prescription:
   a. Must use a child-resistant closure.
   b. May use a non-child-resistant closure if authorized by the patient.
   c. Must affix a federal transfer label to the prescription vial.
   d. Must file C-II hard-copy prescriptions separately.
   e. Answers a and b
   f. Answers b and c
   g. Answers b and d
   h. Answers a and e
   i. All of the above apply.

6. Suppose that a patient is injured after taking a medication in the wrong dosage. Also suppose that you, the pharmacist, realized the error and informed the physician who wrote the prescription about the problem. Further suppose that the physician told you to "just fill the prescription," and you did. If the patient sued, the courts would

take issue with the pharmacist due to a concept in the Federal Controlled Substances Act called:
a. Professional accountability
b. Co-liability
c. Corresponding responsibility
d. Negligence
e. Tort suit

7. Which of the following is/are *not* required to appear on a prescription for phenobarbital?
a. Federal legend
b. Expiration dates
c. DEA number
d. Answers a and b
e. Answers b and c

8. If the prescription in the case was written, "Give Bowser the Beagle (a dog) one tablet every 6 hours for pain," and was also called into the pharmacy by an assistant to Bowser's veterinarian, the pharmacist who received the prescription could legally fill and dispense it as an emergency situation.
a. True, the federal CSA does not differentiate between human or animal prescriptions for emergency situations.
b. True, the federal CSA allows agents of prescribers to telephone prescription orders into pharmacies regardless of whether they are for humans, animals, emergencies, or otherwise.
c. False, the federal CSA does not permit pharmacists to dispense prescriptions for animals even in an emergency situation.
d. False, the federal CSA does not permit agents of prescribers to telephone prescription orders into pharmacies regardless of whether they are for humans, animals, emergencies, or otherwise.
e. Answers a and b are true.

Answers

1d. The federal Controlled Substances Act permits pharmacists to fill prescriptions in an emergency situation provided that the patient's medical condition requires immediate treatment and a CII controlled substance only, and the prescriber is unable to give the patient a hard-copy prescription. Physicians have 7 days in which to mail a hard-copy prescription to the pharmacy that dispensed the emergency prescription.

2c. Correct DEA registration numbers are determined by a formula. Practitioners will have the letter "A" or "B" in the first alpha position followed by the first letter of their last names. Wholesalers and other distributors will have the letter "R." For pharmacists to verify if a DEA registration number on a prescription is correct, the formula is as follows:

> First: Add digits 1, 3, and 5 and determine a sum
> Second: Add digits 2, 4, and 6, determine a sum, and multiply this by 2
> Third: Add both sums, the second digit of this sum (called the "check-digit") equals the last digit of the DEA registration number

3e. Oral prescription orders for controlled substances in Schedule II require hard-copy prescriptions mailed or sent to the dispensing pharmacy within 7 days. Schedules III–V do not.

4e. Pharmacies are permitted under federal regulation to accept prescription orders via facsimile and maintain the faxed copy as an original hard copy provided the patient is medically diagnosed as terminally ill, in hospice care, on intravenous medications, or is in a long-term care facility.

5e. When pharmacists dispense any prescription, regardless of federal schedule, that pharmacist must affix a child-resistant closure unless authorized by the patient to do otherwise or when dispensing an exempt medication such as nitroglycerine SL tablets. A federal transfer label must also be affixed to any prescription container when dispensing federally controlled substances in Schedules II–IV. All prescriptions for CII controlled substances must be kept in a file separate from other prescriptions for controlled substances.

6c. Pharmacists are responsible for the prescriptions they fill that are not for a legitimate medical purpose and are not in the usual course of professional practice.

7c. All prescriptions for controlled substances require the DEA registration number of the prescriber be placed on that prescription to be complete.

8e. The federal CSA does not address the types of prescriptions that may be called into pharmacies in emergency situations unless they are for drugs in Schedule II. The Act does permit agents of prescribers to telephone all prescriptions into pharmacies.

Case #2

A pharmacist takes over a pharmacy in June of a given year. That pharmacist applies for and is granted a DEA registration for the pharmacy. Later, the pharmacist realizes that she needs to take an inventory of all federally controlled substances. After taking this inventory, she finds that she is short significant quantities of several controlled substances. She reports the shortage to DEA and takes appropriate measures to prevent this from happening again.

Questions

1. A DEA Form-222 is used when:
   a. Pharmacists want to borrow CIIIs from other pharmacies.

   b. A theft or loss of controlled substances occurs.
   c. Pharmacists want to order more books of order forms.
   d. Pharmacists want to destroy controlled substances.
   e. None of the above statements is true.
 2. Which of the following is true regarding the federal law on controlled substances inventories.
   a. Inventories for controlled substances in Schedules III and IV, regardless of original quantity in the stock bottle, must be counted exactly.
   b. Inventories for controlled substances must be taken at least once every 2 years from the initial inventory date.
   c. Inventories for controlled substances should be taken every other year (biennially) and may be changed after prior notification to DEA.
   d. Answers a and b are true.
   e. Answers a and c are true.
 3. Under federal laws and regulations, if a pharmacist is granted a Power of Attorney by a registrant, that pharmacist may:
   a. Sign all legal documents that concern the pharmacy
   b. Practice pharmacy law
   c. Open and manage other pharmacies
   d. Sign DEA Form-222 to order controlled substances in Schedule II
   e. Become the manager for the pharmacy
 4. A DEA Form-106 is used when:
   a. Pharmacists want to borrow CIIIs from other pharmacies.
   b. A theft or loss of federally controlled substances occurs.
   c. Pharmacists want to order more books of order forms.
   d. Pharmacists want to destroy controlled substances.
   e. None of the above statements is true.
 5. A DEA Form-41 is used when:
   a. Pharmacists want to borrow CIIIs from other pharmacies.
   b. A theft or loss of federally controlled substances occurs.
   c. Pharmacists want to order more books of order forms.
   d. Pharmacists want to destroy controlled substances.
   e. None of the above statements is true.

 Answers

1e. DEA Form-222 is used when a DEA registrant wishes to order controlled substances in Schedules I and II for stock.

2b. DEA permits its registrants to take an inventory of federally controlled substances at any time within the 2 calendar years of the initial inventory.

3d. A pharmacist granted a Power of Attorney by a registrant is permitted by DEA to sign DEA Form-222 to order controlled substances in Schedule II for pharmacy stock.

4b.   DEA Form-106 is used when a DEA registrant is required to report a theft or a significant loss of federally controlled substances has occurred.

5d.   A DEA Form-41 is used when a DEA registrant wishes to remove unused, expired, or damaged controlled substances from inventory.

Case #3

John, the pharmacist, receives a prescription from Mr. Thomas Hall. He is spending some time with his family in another state. The prescription is for an oral diabetic medication that he uses to treat his diabetes. He writes in separate cover letter, "Please mail out a few refills worth and send me a bill with the medication." You check his patient profile and realize that the dosage prescribed is different from what he had been using. You telephone the doctor who states that Mr. Hall's diabetes has indeed gotten worse, hence the change in the prescription. The prescription is then filled and mailed per the patient's request.

Questions

1. According to U.S. Postal Regulations, which of the following filled prescriptions can be mailed to ultimate users?
   a. Diabetes medication
   b. Glaucoma medication
   c. Narcotics
   d. Answers a and b only can be mailed
   e. All of the above
2. A short time after the hard copy of the prescription for the diabetes medication was mailed to you, Mr. Hall calls your pharmacy to request that you also send him whatever quantity is left on the remaining refills of his CIV narcotic-containing medication. Again, you check his computer profile and find two refills remain. However, the last time he refilled this prescription was 7 months ago. Under *federal law*, what should you do?
   a. Do not refill the prescription. Prescriptions for Schedule IV drugs are valid for five refills or 6 months, whichever is earlier.
   b. Fill the prescription only for the quantity written on the face of the prescription, take it to the nearest U.S. post office, and mail it to the patient.
   c. Fill the prescription with the quantity of the remaining refills, take it to the nearest U.S. post office, and mail it to the patient.
   d. Answers b and c.
   e. All of the above actions are illegal under federal law.
3. Which of the following statements is/are false with regard to U.S. Postal Regulations?
   a. Pharmacists cannot mail filled prescriptions for narcotics listed in Schedule II.

    b. Pharmacists must clearly label all outer packages containing filled prescriptions with the name and address of the pharmacy.

    c. Pharmacists need not label the inner container of a mailed package as long as that container has a child-resistant closure.

    d. Pharmacists cannot mail filled prescriptions listed in Schedule III to ultimate users.

    e. All of the above are false statements.

4. Mr. Hall was in the care of a number of health professionals. Which of the following would not be considered a practitioner?

    a. Allopathic physician

    b. Psychologist

    c. Psychiatrist

    d. Podiatrist

    e. Dentist

5. Pharmacists may lawfully fill prescriptions written by medical interns or foreign physicians when:

    a. They are assigned a suffix to be used with the institutional (i.e., hospital) DEA registration number.

    b. They are assigned a prefix to be used with the institutional (i.e., hospital) DEA registration number.

    c. They write prescriptions that are then co-signed by the chief of residency or other authorized practitioner within the institution.

    d. Answers a and c are correct.

    e. Answers b and c are correct.

6. Which of the following statements is/are true regarding a prescription for a controlled substance?

    a. Written in ink

    b. Written in indelible pencil

    c. Typewritten

    d. Signed by the prescriber in his or her own handwriting

    e. All of the above

7. The federal Controlled Substances Act limits prescription refills of up to five times within 6 months for:

    a. Emergency CII prescriptions only

    b. Telephoned CIII, IV, and V prescriptions only

    c. Any CII, III, and IV prescriptions with authorized refills

    d. Any CIII and IV prescriptions with authorized refills

    e. All prescriptions

Answers

1e. U.S. Postal Regulations permit the mailing of any filled prescription for any controlled substance in any quantity.

2a. Schedule IV prescriptions may not be filled after five refills or 6 months from their date of issue.

3e. All are false.

4b. A psychologist is a Ph.D. who is specially trained to treat mental illness through counseling and is not eligible under federal law to obtain a DEA registration; therefore, a psychologist is not considered to be a practitioner. However, some states may, based on their laws, permit psychologists to have limited prescribing authority as mid-level prescribers. The other professionals are considered to be practitioners under the CSA. A psychiatrist is an M.D. whose specialty is the medical treatment of mental illness; an allopathic physician is by general definition an M.D. who practices any specialty in conventional medicine, i.e., dermatology, internal medicine, oncology, cardiology; a dentist is a specialist in the medical treatment of the teeth and mouth; and a podiatrist is a specialist in the medical treatment of the feet.

5a. Pharmacists may lawfully fill prescriptions written by medical interns or foreign physicians when they are assigned a suffix to be used with the institutional (i.e., hospital) DEA registration number. No co-signature is required.

6e. According to federal law, a prescription for a controlled substance must be written in ink or indelible pencil or typewritten, and signed by the prescriber in his or her own handwriting.

7d. The federal Controlled Substances Act limits prescription refills of up to five times within 6 months for any CIII and IV prescriptions with authorized refills.

Case #4

Your pharmacy's fax machine in buzzing; you can hardly keep the paper supply full. Most of the transmissions are from your state pharmacy association with information on proposed legislation. Continuing education (CE) providers are letting you know about their new programs and a few are even prescriptions. One such prescription is from Dr. Reginald Foote, a noted orthopedic surgeon in your area. He faxes a prescription for Bill Donovan, one of your patients and an avid hiker. The prescription is for oxycodone and acetaminophen tablets, #30, one tablet two or three times daily for ankle fracture. A few hours later, Mr. Donovan comes hobbling into your pharmacy on crutches and asks for his prescription. You have it ready and ask for the hard copy from the physician. He tells you that he never took it from the doctor because he saw the secretary fax it to you. You explain that by law you cannot give him the medication unless he has the original. He angrily shouts, "I saw her fax it, I want my medication; why do you always make it so hard for people?"

Questions

1. Under federal law, which of the following is/are true?
    a. Only patients who have a terminal illness may have prescriptions faxed into a pharmacy.

    b. Patients who are ambulatory and living at home may have pre-scriptions faxed into a pharmacy.

    c. Patients who are ambulatory and living at home may have CII prescriptions faxed into the pharmacy provided they bring the original hard copy with them when they come to pick them up.

    d. Answers a and b are correct.

    e. Answers b and c are correct.

2. If Mr. Donovan's prescription was for acetaminophen with codeine, 30 mg, which would be true?

    a. The pharmacy still could not dispense it to the patient unless a hard copy was brought in.

    b. The pharmacy could dispense it and use the fax as the hard copy.

    c. The pharmacy can only keep faxed prescriptions as hard copy if they are for medications in Schedules IV and V.

    d. The pharmacist cannot, under federal law, accept any faxed pre-scriptions for controlled substances.

    e. The faxed prescription can only be filled for a quantity not to exceed a 7-day supply.

3. If Mr. Donovan, in your professional judgment, needed some medi-cation immediately, what could you do without violating federal law?

    a. Call the physician and request an emergency supply of a few tablets (and a hard-copy back-up) until the hard copy for the original quantity is received by you.

    b. Give the patient a few tablets, void the remainder, and call the physician to request a hard-copy back-up for the tablets that you dispensed.

    c. Give the patient a few tablets, and instruct him to get the hard copy from the physician before any further quantity would be dispensed to him.

    d. Answers a and b are correct.

    e. Answers b and c are correct.

Answers

1e. Patients who are ambulatory and living at home may have any pre-scription faxed into a pharmacy. CII prescriptions may be faxed and filled as a convenience to the patient; however, patients must bring the original hard copy with them when they pick up the medications.

2b. Pharmacies may keep the faxed copy as the hard copy for any pre-scription in Schedules III–V that is faxed to them.

3d. Federal law allows a pharmacist to make certain professional judg-ments. In this case, if Mr. Donovan could not get back to the physi-cian, the pharmacist could, in the best interest of the patient, call the physician and explain the situation. If the physician agrees, the phar-macist could then dispense an emergency supply, void the remaining quantity, and request a hard copy to cover the quantity dispensed.

If the patient needed more CII medication, he would have to bring a hard copy to the pharmacist for dispensing.

Case #5

Many of the telephone calls that come into a busy pharmacy are for new prescriptions. Several of those are from people who work for a physician rather than from the physician himself. One day, you receive a strange call. It is from a local physician's office from which prescriptions are received many times daily; however, the caller is unfamiliar to you and seems to be unsure of the prescription. It is for a CIV anti-anxiety medication for a patient who is also new to you. You question the caller and ask if she works for the physician and she tells you, "Not usually, I'm just filling in for a few hours because the secretary has the flu." She then tells you that the doctor gave her a whole bunch of prescriptions to call into various pharmacies in the city while he goes to the hospital to see a patient. What should you do?

Questions

1. In this case, based on federal law and corresponding responsibility, the pharmacist should just fill the prescription.
   a. True
   b. False
2. In this case, who would be permitted to call new prescriptions into a pharmacy for a controlled substance.
   a. A secretary
   b. A nurse
   c. A clerk
   d. A delivery man
   e. Any of the above who act at the direction of the physician
3. What should the pharmacist do if he or she decides to fill the prescription?
   a. Write the name of the person who called the prescription into the pharmacy on its face.
   b. Request a hard copy be sent within 7 days.
   c. Make sure that the prescription is complete and all required information is present.
   d. Answers a and b are correct.
   e. Answers a and c are correct.

Answers

1b. In cases where the pharmacist believes that a prescription may be incorrect, the pharmacist must make the effort to validate it with the physician. The best approach would be to page the physician at the hospital or wait until the physician has returned to the office to verify the prescription as correct.

2e. Anyone who is acting on behalf of the physician and is directed by the physician to call in a prescription may do so. One might prefer another type of medical personnel such as nurse or physician assistant, but a secretary, clerk, or delivery person may as well.

3e. If the pharmacist decides to fill this prescription, he or she would need to have all the required information on the telephone order as well as the name of the person who transmitted the prescription.

OBRA '90

Case #6

Charles Spivak, a senior college student and co-captain of the varsity basketball team, enters the campus pharmacy to fill a new prescription for an albuterol inhaler for his asthma. The pharmacist informs Charlie that this medication will cost just over $20.00 and should last approximately 2 to 3 weeks with proper use. Charles, knowing that he needs some form of medication so that he will be able to play in the upcoming playoffs, asks Karen, the pharmacist, if there are any over-the-counter alternatives. Karen explains to Charles that his medication has numerous advantages over the nonprescription asthmatic medications including increased effectiveness, safety, and a lower incidence of side effects. She counsels Charles on the medication's proper use and reviews its advantages over other medications. After hearing this, he is reassured that this prescription is right for him.

Questions

1. Under federal OBRA '90 regulations, which of the following would be considered a legal offer to counsel?
   a. Telephone communication with the patient
   b. An auxiliary label on a prescription vial
   c. A toll-free telephone number
   d. A sign posted informing customers of the right to counseling
   e. A cartoon illustration demonstrating how to take a medication for patients who do not speak English
   f. Answers a, b, and c
   g. Answers b, c, and d
   h. Answers c, d, and e
   i. Answers a, c, and d
   j. Answers b and d

2. Federal OBRA '90 regulations require the offer to counsel be given to:
   a. All patients for both new and refill prescriptions
   b. Medicaid patients, and only for new prescriptions
   c. All patients on new prescriptions
   d. Medicaid patients for both new and refill prescriptions
   e. None of the above

3. Which of the following is/are true?
   a. OBRA '90 is actually the mnemonic for the Federal Budget of the United States of America.
   b. With regard to pharmacy and OBRA '90, the piece of legislation that has caused professional hoopla is called the Medicaid Prudent Pharmaceutical Purchasing Act.
   c. OBRA '90 deals primarily with community pharmacy practice.
   d. All of the above are true.
4. Which statements are true regarding OBRA '90.
   a. OBRA '90 legislation spells out what pharmacists are expected to do within the context of the healthcare system.
   b. OBRA will help the courts decide whether or not a pharmacist "did something" properly or not.
   c. The idea that pharmacists can "do something" as a benefit to healthcare is not new.
   d. All of the above are true.

Answers

1d. Pharmacists may call patients to offer counseling if the person receiving the prescription is not the patient, may give a toll-free telephone number, or may post a sign offering counseling.
2d. Federal OBRA '90 regulations require pharmacists to offer counseling to Medicaid patients only. States may impose their own requirements.
3d. All of the above are true.
4d. All of the above are true.

Case #7

Mary Belker is a seventh grader who does a lot for her mother. She helps around the house and does her chores. Mary feels that she is important to the family because her mother has a chronic pulmonary condition that prevents her from being as active as she would like. One of Mary's jobs is to go to the pharmacy and pick up her mother's prescriptions. She knows how hard her mother struggles to go to work to support her and her brother and when she sees how expensive her mother's medication is, she asks the pharmacist if it is really worth the cost or will other pills do the same thing? She asks the pharmacist if there is anything that she should tell her mother. She appears somewhat puzzled about the medication but wants to help her mother. The pharmacist assures her that the drug helps control the progress of the disease and is the very best medical option to allow her mother to continue to do the many things that she does. "Without the drug," the pharmacist told her, "the disease would confine your mother to bed."

Questions

1. OBRA requires pharmacists to obtain, record, and maintain all of the following except:
   a. Patient disease state

    b. List of drug medications

    c. Relevant medical devices

    d. Method of payment

2. Under OBRA, a pharmacist will need to interact with a prescriber on behalf of a patient on issues which may include

    a. Therapeutic duplication

    b. Drug–drug interaction

    c. Drug–disease interaction

    d. All of the above are true

3. In the above case, how should the pharmacist counsel the patient properly if she accepts?

    a. Counsel the 12-year-old daughter.

    b. Call the mother and ask her if she has any questions.

    c. Write or print the information onto paper and send it home with the prescription.

    d. Answers a and b are true.

    e. Answers b and c are true.

4. In Massachusetts, which of the following is/are true?

    a. Pharmacists *must* provide all existing medical information to patients.

    b. Pharmacists may use their professional judgment regarding the information provided to the patient.

    c. Pharmacists may delegate the actual counseling to pharmacy technicians who are well trained and are certified.

    d. Patients may be given written information which is then considered complete counseling with no further responsibilities to the pharmacist.

Answers

1d. OBRA does not require that pharmacists obtain, record, and maintain a patient's method of payment.

2d. Pharmacists must conduct a prospective drug use review (DUR) to ensure optimum therapeutic outcomes.

3e. Pharmacists can counsel patients by telephone or by using written communication provided patients understand that this written communication is not complete and further questions should be addressed to the pharmacist.

4b. Pharmacists may use their professional judgment regarding how much information they provide to the patient. A pharmacist's counseling should be complete and care should be taken to include all of the most common side effects, adverse effects, and warnings.

Product selection

Case #8

Earl Tibbitts, 74, was perplexed. His wife Laura is 72 years old and has had many urinary tract infections. Each time they see the doctor, he tells Laura that she has that infection again and gives her a prescription for a different antibiotic. Each time they get the prescription for the new antibiotic filled at the pharmacy, the price rises. Earl asks if the stuff is made of gold. The pharmacist tells him that the new product may just do the trick. "After all," the pharmacist says, "this prescription has only once-daily dosing instead of four times daily as with the other drugs. And, ease and convenience are only part of the benefit, this particular medication has been designed to combat resistant organisms such as the one that has been troubling your wife so much." "Thank goodness," said Earl, "the doctor said that if the problem didn't get fixed, he'd put Laura in the hospital for more intense therapy and with our insurance, we're still trying to pay for the last hospitalization." Earl then asks if it comes in a "genetic" form. You smile and tell him that since the product is so new, it doesn't have a "generic" equivalent yet. He then asks, "Is there any thing that's close so as I don't have to spend so much money?"

Questions
1. If the drug could be substituted in this case, it would be:
   a. "A" rated.
   b. "B" rated.
   c. "BX" rated.
   d. Answers a and b are correct.
   e. Answers a and c are correct.
2. Which of the following categories is/are *not* listed in the Orange Book?
   a. Generic products not legally interchangeable with products of another company.
   b. "B"-rated drug products
   c. Drugs on patent for which there is no legally interchangeable product.
   d. Answers a and b are correct.
   e. Answers a and c are correct.
3. A drug product that is given an A rating in the FDA "Approved Drugs with Therapeutic Equivalence Evaluations" would be officially characterized by FDA as:
   a. Pharmacotherapeutic
   b. Bioavailable
   c. Therapeutically equivalent
   d. Bioequivalent
   e. Pharmaceutically equivalent

Answers
1a. An A-rated product is considered by FDA to be therapeutically equivalent in its rate and extent of absorption and distribution.
2c. The Orange Book lists only those products for which an off patent or multisource drug is available. Therefore, if a product is off patent

and is only available from one manufacturer due to the expense of manufacture or low consumer demand, it will not be listed. If a product is new to the marketplace and on patent with no generic version available, it also will not be listed.

3c. Though an A-rated drug will have all of the components listed in the answer key, the official designation, therapeutic equivalence encompasses all of them because a product must certainly be pharmacotherapeutic and bioavailable to the body's physiology. In addition, the definition of a therapeutically equivalent drug product is that it is bioequivalent (to the pioneer product with a similar rate and extent of absorption, distribution, excretion, etc.) and pharmaceutically equivalent in that it is the same dose and dosage form as well.

Food, Drug and Cosmetic Act

Case #9

Your pharmacy receives a letter from a pharmaceutical manufacturer which states that it is conducting a recall of a certain product because of reports that the tablets are breaking up in the stock bottle during shipment resulting in many unusable doses. The letter also states that the problem is not dangerous to patients in any way. You check your pharmacy shelves and find that you have two stock bottles on the shelf. One has been opened and has had tablets dispensed from it. Luckily, the other bottle is unopened and has the lot number of the product that has been recalled printed on its label. You remove this recalled product and prepare to send it back to the manufacturer. However, you notice that the opened bottle appears to be within 3 months of its expiration date. You remembered that you had just opened it the other day to make a few "bingo cards" or blister packs for a nursing home patient who you service. These cards of medication have not yet been delivered to the nursing home and you wonder if your technician has used the proper expiration date on their labels. You check the order and find that they have been labeled properly.

Questions

1. How would you characterize this incident?
    a. Class I, consumer level
    b. Class II, consumer level
    c. Class II, retail level
    d. Class III, retail level
    e. Class III, consumer level
2. There are federal regulations regarding expiration dating on a manufacturer's stock bottle based on stability of product as packaged and as stored by the manufacturer. However, in products that are very

stable, i.e., dry powders and capsules, what is the federal requirement for product expiration date?
   a.   5 years
   b.   7 years
   c.   10 years
   d.   2 years
   e.   None of the above
3.   What is the United States Pharmacopeia's (USP) recommendation for expiration dating on a prescription label when a drug is dispensed from a community retail pharmacy?
   a.   The date on the manufacturer's stock bottle
   b.   6 months from the date dispensed
   c.   1 year from the date dispensed
   d.   Answer a or b, whichever is earlier
   e.   Answer a or c, whichever is earlier
4.   The proper expiration dating used when hospital pharmacies repackage medications into unit-doses is:
   a.   25% of the time remaining of the date on the manufacturer's stock bottle
   b.   6 months from the date repackaged
   c.   1 year from the date repackaged
   d.   Answer a or b, whichever is earlier
   e.   Answer a or c, whichever is earlier
5.   The proper expiration date used on insulin products is:
   a.   Until any date that the manufacturer proves the product is stable
   b.   6 months from the date manufactured
   c.   1 year from the date manufactured
   d.   2 years from the date manufactured
   e.   None of the above

Answers

1d.   Recalls are not under the statutory authority of the FDA. However, it can recommend that a company recall a product from the marketplace if the product is under FDA jurisdiction and if that product in some way jeopardizes the health and safety of the public. Companies whose products are under FDA jurisdiction and are a danger to the health of the public may recall these products at any time. Class I recalls indicate grave danger or possible irreversible threat to public safety, i.e., may cause death or grave bodily injury if ingested. Class II recalls indicate a public safety threat, but one which is reversible or not life-threatening, i.e., may cause fever or vomiting if ingested. Class III recalls indicate no threat to public safety but the product is in some way defective, i.e., butter left out of buttered popcorn. A consumer-level recall indicates that the product in question must be removed from the consumer's home or elsewhere. A retail-level recall indicates that the product in question must be removed from the pharmacy's shelves. A retail-level recall indicates that the product in question must be removed from pharmacy wholesalers or other sites of distribution.

2e.   No federal requirement exists regarding product expiration. Expiration is based on stability studies conducted by manufacturers of products that cover a number of conditions such as packaging and storage.

3e.   USP recommends that prescription labels used when a medication is dispensed from a community retail pharmacy bear an expiration date that is the same as the date on the manufacturer's stock bottle or 1 year from the date the product is dispensed to the patient, whichever is earlier.

4e.   USP recommends that prescription labels used when a medication is dispensed in unit-dose from a hospital or institutional pharmacy bear an expiration date of 25% of the time remaining from the date on the manufacturer's stock bottle or 6 months from the date repackaged, whichever is earlier.

5d.   The proper expiration date used on insulin products is 2 years from the date manufactured.

Case #10

Medical Pharmacy has been a member of a small town community for years. As such, pharmacist owner David Williams belongs to many civic and business organizations. One such organization has a monthly luncheon speaker who may present a topic of his or her choice. David was asked to name a speaker for next month's meeting. He thought long and hard and then remembered attending a recent continuing education program presented by a college of pharmacy faculty member. Her topic was the approval process of prescription drugs in the United States. He thinks several of the members would be intrigued by her comments regarding pricing and reimbursement and how prescription medications "actually get on the market."

Questions

1.   Which of the following is/are false regarding use of the National Drug Code (NDC)?

a.   It is not required by law to be on all product labels for prescription drugs.

b.   It consists of 12 digits. The first set of digits identifies the product.

c.   If a product label has an NDC number on it, one could assume that the product requires a prescription.

d.   Answer a or b is false.

e.   Answer b or c is false.

f.   Answer c only.

g.   Answers a and b only.

h.   Answers b and c only.

2. _____ prohibits pharmacies from storing, dispensing, or purchasing prescription drug samples and requires state boards of pharmacy to license drug wholesalers:
   a. Poison Prevention Packaging Act
   b. Price Competition and Patent Restoration Act
   c. Prescription Drug Marketing Act
   d. Kefauver–Harris Amendments
   e. Food, Drug and Cosmetic Act

3. _____ required the examination of all prescription medications manufactured between 1938 and 1962 to determine drug effectiveness.
   a. Poison Prevention Packaging Act
   b. Price Competition and Patent Restoration Act
   c. Prescription Drug Marketing Act
   d. Kefauver–Harris Amendments
   e. Food, Drug and Cosmetic Act

4. _____ is the largest human testing phase in drug development in which more data on safety and efficacy are gathered through a more diverse test population.
   a. Phase I
   b. Phase II
   c. Phase III
   d. Phase IV
   e. Phase V

5. _____ is the phase where long-term safety, efficacy, and monitoring are established after marketing approval is granted.
   a. Phase I
   b. Phase II
   c. Phase III
   d. Phase IV
   e. Phase V

6. Products that are contaminated after they are shipped to a retail outlet are considered to be _____ but not _____.
   a. Misdirected, inconsistent
   b. Misbranded, adulterated
   c. Adulterated, misbranded
   d. Misbranded, USP
   e. USP, misbranded

7. Manufacturers who wish to add a new indication for a product already being marketed must submit a(n) _____ to FDA for approval of the change.
   a. SNDA
   b. NDA
   c. INDA
   d. ANDA
   e. PANDA

Answers

1e. The National Drug Code consists of an 11-digit code in which the first four digits identify the labeler, the next four digits identify the product, and the last set of two digits identifies the package size. NDC numbers on products labels do not necessarily indicate that the product is a legend or prescription drug.

2c. The Prescription Drug Marketing Act prohibits pharmacies from storing, dispensing, or purchasing prescription drug samples and requires state boards of pharmacy to license drug wholesalers.

3d. The Kefauver–Harris Amendments to the federal Food, Drug and Cosmetic Act required the examination of all prescription medications manufactured between 1938 and 1962 to determine drug effectiveness.

4c. Phase III is the largest human testing phase in drug development for which more data on safety and efficacy are gathered through a more diverse test population.

5d. Phase IV is the phase where long-term safety, efficacy, and monitoring are established after marketing approval is granted.

6c. A product may considered adulterated if it becomes contaminated after it is shipped to a retail outlet. A product may be considered misbranded if its labeling does not reflect the true contents of the container to which it is affixed.

7a. A Supplemental New Drug Application (SNDA) is used by manufacturers who wish to amend an existing NDA to include a new indication, dose form, or manufacturing process.

Prescription Drug Marketing Act

Case #11

One morning the telephone rings in your pharmacy. The caller is a local physician with whom you have a very cordial relationship. He asks if you're still on for golf on Sunday and tells you that he has a deal for you that you just can't refuse. It seems his office staff has been ordering prescription drug samples in fairly large quantities. He sheepishly tells you that he just signed the paperwork for these orders and never gave them much thought. Then yesterday, he wanted a patient to have a few samples of a certain medication to get started and asked his nurse to get them. When she did, she brought several boxes. He asked, "How much of this stuff do we have?" Her answer was "enough to supply a small city!!" He took a look and found thousands of dosage units of medication samples in his storage room. He knows that the cost for all of these samples has to be over $10,000. "Let's make a deal," he says, "give me $1000 and you can have them all."

Questions

1. According to the Prescription Drug Marketing Act, which of the following is/are true?
   a. Pharmacists may purchase prescription drug samples provided they pay fair market price for them.
   b. Pharmacists may purchase prescription drug samples provided they add them to their inventory at the time of purchase.
   c. By federal law pharmacists are prohibited from purchasing and redispensing.
   d. Pharmacists may purchase prescription drug samples and designate them for resale to indigent patients at a reduced price.
   e. Answers a, b, and d are true.
2. Regarding hospital pharmacies and prescription drug samples, which of the following is/are permissible under the Prescription Drug Marketing Act?
   a. Hospital pharmacies may store prescription drug samples provided they are kept separate from other pharmacy stock.
   b. Hospital pharmacies must keep copies of the prescriber's written request to the pharmaceutical company for prescription drug samples.
   c. Hospital pharmacies may not offer prescription drug samples for sale to any individual.
   d. Answers a and c are true.
   e. All of the above are true.
3. Regarding drug wholesalers, which of the following is/are true?
   a. The PDMA requires drug wholesalers to become registered as such by FDA.
   b. The PDMA requires drug wholesalers to become registered as such by the state in which they operate.
   c. The PDMA requirement for registration is voluntary for those drug wholesalers who wish to distribute prescription drug samples.
   d. The PDMA does not include regulatory requirements for drug wholesalers.
   e. All of the above are true.

Answers

1c. One of the major intents of the PDMA was to prevent the diversion of prescription drug samples from a public health as well as law enforcement standpoint. FDA felt that many samples that were expired, damaged, or otherwise adulterated were being sold to pharmacies.
2e. The PDMA was implemented to prevent pharmacies from dispensing or storing samples. However, in many institutional settings, it may be more sensible for the pharmacy to store sample medications in an

effort to better control them. The PDMA permits this activity under certain conditions as listed in the question.

3b.   The PDMA requires drug wholesalers to register with the states in which they operate to better monitor their activities and to prevent diversion.

Mid-level practitioners

Case #12

A new pediatrics group has just moved into your area. As a good neighbor, you call the practice and speak with the pediatrician who owns the practice. You tell her about your services, willingness to be a partner in healthcare, and inquire as to their needs and expectations from a pharmacy. She laughs and tells you that she really hasn't thought about any of that but she's sure that her four nurse practitioners will have some suggestions. She then tells you that she leaves almost all of the prescribing to them. She thanks you for your professional courtesy and hangs up. At this point, you think, "I wonder what I'm in for?"

Questions
1.   Which of the following DEA numbers is correct for Mary Sullivan, a nurse practitioner who practices in your neighborhood?
   a.   NP 1357938
   b.   AS 1211399
   c.   MS 1221384
   d.   SA 3798611
   e.   RS 1256734
2.   If a nurse practitioner or physician assistant is granted broad and independent prescription writing authority by the federal government and is considered a mid-level practitioner, and a certain state decides to limit those privileges, which of the following is/are true?
   a.   Federal law takes precedence in all cases.
   b.   States cannot refuse to permit any regulatory activity granted under the federal law.
   c.   Mid-level prescribers are subject to whichever regulation is more stringent.
   d.   Answers a and b are true.
   e.   Answers b and c are true.
3.   Which of the following are true regarding mid-level practitioners and prescribing privileges?
   a.   Documentation is required by states regarding conditions of pre-scriptive privileges.
   b.   Documentation should be kept readily available for inspection by DEA.

    c. Practice agreements, practice guidelines, and protocols are examples of required documents.

    d. States are given authority by DEA to set educational standards.

    e. All of the above.

Answers

1c. Correct DEA registration numbers are determined by a formula. Mid-level practitioners will have the letter "M" in the first alpha position followed by the first letter of their last name. For pharmacists to verify if a DEA registration number on a prescription is correct, the formula is as follows:

> First: Add digits 1, 3, and 5 and determine a sum.
>
> Second: Add digits 2, 4, and 6, determine a sum and multiply this by 2.
>
> Third: Add both sums, the second digit of this sum (called the "check-digit") equals the last digit of the DEA registration number.

2c. As with all regulations, federal regulations take precedence unless those of a state are more stringent. In this case, DEA allows prescriptive privileges to mid-level prescribers as long as the state in which the person practices allows it as well.

3e. Documentation is required by all mid-level practitioners who are given prescribing privileges by the states. Practice guidelines, agreements, and protocols may be used and must be readily available for inspection by DEA.

Poison Prevention Packaging Act

Case #13

Bill Parsons is an elderly patient with severely arthritic hands. He insists that he get all of his prescriptions without those "damn safety caps." "Too hard to get off by us older folks." "No problem," you say. You add his request for non-child-resistant closures to his patient profile in the computer. Later you wonder, "should I have gotten his request in writing? Bill has quite a lot of grandchildren who visit."

Questions

1. According to the Poison Prevention Packaging Act, which of the following requires complying containers?

    a. Prescription drugs for oral use

    b. Oral contraceptives in mnemonic packages

    c. Potassium supplements less than 50 mEqs

    d. Powdered cholestyramine

    e. Topical creams and ointments

2. Which of the following comply with the requirements for packaging under the Poison Prevention Packaging Act?

    a. Nitroglycerin sublingual tabs in non-child-resistant containers

    b. OTC ibuprofen tablets packaged in clearly marked, non-child-resistant containers of 100 for arthritic elderly patient suspension.

    c. Children's aspirin in child-resistant containers.

    d. Prescription medication packaged in non-child-resistant containers with permission from the patient.

    e All of the above require special packaging.

3. Which of the following is/are true under the PPPA?

    a. Prescriptions dispensed in plastic containers must be discarded and have new containers when dispensing the refill.

    b. Prescriptions dispensed in glass containers must be discarded and have new containers when dispensing the refill.

    c. Patients may verbally request that prescriptions must be dispensed to them in non-child-resistant containers.

    d. Answers a and c are true.

    e. Answers b and c are true.

Answers

1a. All prescription drugs for oral use, unless exempt by regulation, the patient, or physician, must be dispensed in child-resistant containers.

2e. The Poison Prevention Packaging Act permits certain medications to be packaged in non-child-resistant containers, i.e., nitroglycerin. OTC products for elderly arthritic users may also be packaged in containers with non-child-resistant closures that are clearly marked as such and in only one package size.

3b. Prescription refills must be dispensed in new containers if the original filling was dispensed in a plastic container because of the possibility that the locking mechanism may become worn after repeated opening. Prescriptions dispensed in glass containers need only replacement of child-resistant caps. Patients may verbally request that prescriptions be dispensed to them in non-child-resistant containers; however, the Consumer Product Safety Commission recommends that pharmacists obtain a written exemption statement prior to dispensing the medication to the patient in non-child-resistant caps.

Expiration dating and NDC code

Case #14

It's Tuesday morning in your busy hospital pharmacy and your wholesaler delivers your prescription drug order. You ask your technician to put the order away and instruct him to be careful that all drugs are stocked in the right place, behind any opened, existing bottles of the same medication. You also instruct him to check for product expiration dates while he's at it. He replies that he's kind of new to the job and isn't sure he'll know what is really the same. He also asks how close to the bottle's printed expiration date is the guide to remove the product from stock? You explain about NDC numbers and how they are distinct and identify products individually. You also tell him that it's the policy of the hospital pharmacy to remove any product within 30 days of its printed expiration from stock.

Questions

1. Human over-the-counter consumer products (i.e., shampoo, tooth-paste) are exempt from FDA expiration dating regulations if:
   a. They are stable for at least 5 years.
   b. Their labeling bears dosage limitations.
   c. They are safe and effective.
   d. They are safe and suitable for frequent and often prolonged use.
   e. None of the above.
2. If an NDC number is used on a product label by a manufacturer, where must it appear?
   a. The NDC number is required to appear on the top third of the principal display panel of all drug product labels from manufacturers.
   b. The NDC number is required to appear anywhere on the manufacturer's product label.
   c. The NDC number is required to appear on the outer package only.
   d. The NDC number is required to appear on the prescription label.
   e. All of the above.

Answers

1d. Human OTC products that are to be used in a relatively short period of time and are medicated are exempt from FDA expiration dating regulations.
2a. If a manufacturer chooses to use an NDC number on its product labels, the number is required to appear on the top third of the principal display panel of all drug product labels.

Over-the-counter drugs

Case #15

Mr. Tom Maher telephones the pharmacy to request a refill on his arthritis medicine. Something, call it intuition, tells you to check his profile. You tell him to hold on while you check. AHA!!! Just as you've suspected, no valid refills are left. You tell Mr. Maher that you'll contact his physician and deliver the prescription after you get proper authorization. He thanks you and hangs up. You call his physician and request the new prescription. The physician's nurse looks at the patient record and realizes that Mr. Maher hasn't been in to see the doctor for at least 18 months. She asks the physician about refilling the medication and he says, "NO ... Tell him to see me." You call the patient and relay the news. The patient says that the doctor costs too much ... the drug he needs is OTC anyway, he'll just triple the dose to equal the prescription strength.

Questions

1. Which of the following is/are false regarding OTC medications?
    a. OTC product labels must by written in understandable language and provide information necessary for safe and effective use by consumers.
    b. OTC products must be appropriate for use by patients only for acute conditions that consumers may identify after professional supervision.
    c. OTC products by design do not require consumers to read the label to use them appropriately.
    d. Answers a and b.
    e. Answers b and c.
2. It could be generally said of the OTC drug review process that:
    a. It allows a company to put new products on the market.
    b. It requires a company to use only those ingredients and their combinations as described by the monograph for that product category.
    c. It permits scientific and public comment about OTC product categories and their ingredients and combinations.
    d. Answers a and b are correct.
    e. Answers b and c are correct.
3. Regarding drugs considered for a switch from RX to OTC status, which of the following is/are true?
    a. Switching RX products to OTC products does not require conducting an entire review process on the product such as submission of a brand new NDA, animal testing, human testing, etc.
    b. The monograph process can be used to facilitate an RX to OTC switch.
    c. The monograph system can be used only when the product can be demonstrated as safe to use by the consumer.
    d. Answers a and b are correct.
    e. Answers b and c are correct.
4. Which of the following criteria is/are used by FDA to classify drugs as having prescription status?
    a. Habit-forming drugs are assigned to prescription status.
    b. Drugs that require a physician's supervision are assigned to prescription status.

   c. Homeopathic drugs with are diluted to "1X" are assigned to prescription status.

   d. Answers a and b apply to FDA criteria for prescription status.

   e. Answers b and c apply to FDA criteria for prescription status.

Answers

1e. OTC product labels must by written in understandable language and provide information necessary for safe and effective use by consumers who are then expected to medicate themselves without intervention by a physician.

2d. The OTC drug review process ultimately gives companies a boilerplate to consult when developing OTC products for market. It permits scientific and public comments about OTC product categories, their ingredients and combinations.

3d. The monograph process, as well as the use of a petition or a supplemental NDA, can be used to facilitate an RX to OTC switch.

4d. The criteria used by FDA to classify drugs as having prescription status include whether the product was shown to be habit forming while in clinical trials or whether the drugs require a physician's supervision for proper use.

part three

Exam review questions

chapter eight

Study questions

1. The _____ requires that pharmacists offer to counsel caregivers who wish to fill new prescriptions for Medicaid patients.
   a. Omnibus Budget Reconciliation Act
   b. Price Competition and Patent Restoration Act
   c. Prescription Drug Marketing Act
   d. Kefauver–Harris Amendments
   e. Food, Drug and Cosmetic Act

2. The _____ mandates that prescription drug samples must be requested by licensed practitioners in writing and that records must be kept documenting which patients receive them.
   a. Omnibus Budget Reconciliation Act
   b. Price Competition and Patent Restoration Act
   c. Prescription Drug Marketing Act
   d. Kefauver–Harris Amendments
   e. Federal Prescription Drug and Sampling Act

3. The _____ permits a corporate tax write-off or deduction to pharmaceutical companies who develop lifesaving drugs for rare diseases or are otherwise unprofitable.
   a. Federal Prescription Drug and Sampling Act
   b. Price Competition and Patent Restoration Act
   c. Prescription Drug Marketing Act
   d. Orphan Drug Act
   e. Food, Drug and Cosmetic Act

4. The _____ mandated the use of NDAs so that pharmaceutical companies had to prove that their drug products were safe.
   a. Federal Prescription Drug and Sampling Act
   b. Price Competition and Patent Restoration Act
   c. Prescription Drug Marketing Act
   d. Orphan Drug Act
   e. Food, Drug and Cosmetic Act

5. Please select the proper answer that lists an example of one controlled substance in each category, CI to CV. These drugs are not necessarily in any particular order.
   a. Tylenol with codeine elixir, Tylenol with codeine tablets, Valium, Percocet, Xanax
   b. Marijuana, Ritalin, Seconal, Halcion, Phenergan with codeine syrup
   c. Marijuana, Percocet, Ritalin, Tylenol with codeine tablets, Tylenol with codeine elixir
   d. Marijuana, Seconal, Valium, Tylenol with codeine tablets, Tylenol with codeine elixir
   e. Dilaudid, Percodan, Xanax, Ativan, Phenergan with codeine syrup

6. If a prescription drug becomes newly controlled or is placed in a more restrictive schedule, the pharmacist must:
   a. Wait until the next scheduled biennial inventory in order to add it to the existing inventory.
   b. Immediately inventory all controlled substances.
   c. Add it to the existing inventory on the official date of rescheduling.
   d. Return all unused portions of the drug to the manufacturer to exchange them for properly labeled products that have a "C" and the new schedule number written in Roman numerals.
   e. Ask prescribers to reissue new prescriptions for patients who are using that particular drug product.

7. If a pharmacist takes an inventory and finds that she is 378 tablets short of morphine sulfate tablets 15 mg, that pharmacist should:
   a. Fill out a DEA Form-222 in triplicate and send one copy to the Board of Pharmacy
   b. Fill out a DEA Form-41 and report the loss to the FDA
   c. Report the loss to the DEA, conduct an inventory of all controlled substances, and then fill out a DEA Form-41 in triplicate.
   d. Report the loss to the local police, conduct an inventory of all controlled substances, and then fill out DEA Form-106 in triplicate.
   e. Call the Board of Pharmacy, ask for a controlled substances audit, and fill out a DEA Form-222a in triplicate.

8. Interns, residents, and foreign physicians are required to have their own personal DEA registration number along with a suffix assigned to them by the hospital with which they are affiliated.
   a. True
   b. False

9. Which of the following Schedules do not require refills to be retrievable by a pharmacy computer system?
   a. CIII
   b. CIV
   c. CV

      d. Answers a and b

      e. Answers b and c

10. Partial dispensing of Schedule III controlled substances requires that:

      a. Pharmacists must dispense all outstanding quantities within 72 hours.

      b. Pharmacists document, either by computer or on the back of the hard copy, the quantity dispensed, the date, and their initials.

      c. Pharmacists determine how many refills will remain after this one is dispensed.

      d. The prescriber is informed that a partial refill has occurred.

      e. None of the above.

11. Current, complete, and accurate records for controlled substances include:

      a. Hard-copy prescriptions that have been previously filled

      b. The third copy of a DEA Form-222

      c. Invoices for drugs ordered in CIII–CV

      d. Answers b and c

      e. All of the above except d

12. All inventories and records for CII must be:

      a. Maintained with other federally controlled substances

      b. Maintained for a period of at least 3 years

      c. Maintained separately from all other controlled substances

      d. Copied in triplicate and submitted to DEA biennially

      e. Copied and kept on file until re-registration with DEA

13. If a registered pharmacist is permitted by DEA to sign DEA Form-222, that pharmacist:

      a. Could be the registrant

      b. Could have power of attorney

      c. Must register with DEA, in writing, with an official signature

      d. Answers a and b

      e. Answers b and c

14. If a veterinarian writes a prescription for a human child and supplies written documentation of medical diagnosis and all diagnostic testing as well as an official prescription, the pharmacist must:

      a. Fill the prescription as written.

      b. Verify the prescription with the practitioner and then fill it.

      c. Require a copy of her DEA registration be on file at the pharmacy.

      d. Fill the prescription for its original quantity with no further refills.

      e. None of the above.

15. When a patient brings a prescription into the pharmacy for tylenol with codeine elixir and asks that you hold it until needed, it is legal for you to do this. However, if that prescription is not filled for 8 or 10 months and the patient calls to request that you fill it, you are legally required to:

      a. Tell the patient that the prescription is too old and that the patient must go to the doctor to get a new one.

   b. Call the patient's physician and request an updated or more recent hard copy.
   c. Fill the prescription.
   d. Answers b and c.
   e. None of the above.

16. The major difference between partially filling a prescription for percocet vs. valium is that:
   a. Percocet may not have its remaining quantity dispensed after 72 hours.
   b. Valium may not have its remaining quantity dispensed after 72 hours.
   c. Valium may not have its remaining quantity dispensed after 7 days.
   d. Valium may have its remaining quantity filled for up to 60 days in a long-term care facility.
   e. Percocet may not have its remaining quantity dispensed after 7 days.

17. Hypothetical: A physician calls your pharmacy by telephone in the middle of a terrible winter ice storm and asks that you fill a prescription for his patient for percocet as an emergency supply. You know that the patient is in a wheelchair, has no family, has bone cancer pain, and is currently connected to antibiotic IV drugs and cannot leave the house. Under federal law,
   a. This situation is in compliance with all of the guidelines for an emergency situation under the CSA and should be filled.
   b. This situation is not in compliance with the guidelines for an emergency situation under the CSA and should not be filled.
   c. This situation is in compliance with some but not all of the guidelines for an emergency situation under the CSA and should not be filled.

18. DEA registrants, such as pharmacies and physicians, who store controlled substances are required to conduct an inventory of:
   a. CIIs at least annually
   b. All federally controlled substances at least biannually
   c. All federally controlled substances at least biennially
   d. All drugs within the premises
   e. All federally controlled substances perpetually (every time product is dispensed to a patient)

19. One could say that the federal requirement for conducting an inventory for CIII controlled substances that the pharmacy buys in bottles of 500 tablets allows pharmacists to guess the total quantity of tablets on hand and in the pharmacy.
   a. True
   b. False

20. Which of the following information is required to appear on a prescription label for CV drugs under federal law?

a. The prescriber's DEA registration number
b. The Federal Transfer label
c. The date filled
d. The number of authorized refills remaining of the prescription
e. The pharmacist's initials

21. Which of the following statements is/are true?
    a. When telephoning an emergency prescription order for a CIII into a pharmacy, a physician has 72 hours to mail the hard copy to the pharmacy for the telephoned prescription.
    b. An emergency veterinary prescription for five percocet tablets (directions: Give Fluffy the cat one half tablet every 8 hours for pain) may only be called in to a pharmacy by a veterinarian.

22. A computerized, automated system used to fill prescriptions must be capable of printing out a hard copy of the current prescription refill activity for Schedules III and IV.
    a. I only
    b. II only
    c. III only
    d. I and II
    e. All of the above

23. The federal CSA limits refills of up to 5 times or within 6 months for:
    a. Emergency CII RXs only
    b. Telephoned CIII, IV, and V RXs only
    c. Any CII, III, and IV RXs with authorization
    d. Any CIII and IV RXs with authorized refills
    e. None of the above

24. The federal Controlled Substances Act requires that pharmacies keep prescriptions on file for:
    a. One (1) year
    b. Two (2) years
    c. Five (5) years
    d. Ten (10) years
    e. An indefinite time period

25. Every pharmacy must re-register with the U.S. DEA if licensed in the United States,
    a. Annually
    b. Biannually
    c. Biennially
    d. Triennially
    e. No registration needed

26. Under the provisions of the Poison Prevention Packaging Act, when a prescription for an oral medication is dispensed in a glass container, the pharmacist:
    a. Must use an entirely new container
    b. May reuse the entire container
    c. May reuse the container and replace the cap

d. May reuse the cap and replace the container

27. According to the Poison Prevention Packaging Act, which of the following requires complying containers?
    a. Prescription drugs for oral use
    b. Oral contraceptives in mnemonic packages
    c. Potassium supplements in unit dose
    d. Aspirin tablets in quantities of 100 if labeled for arthritic use
    e. Topical hydrocortisone cream in >2.5% concentration

28. According to the Poison Prevention Packaging Act, a prescriber can check a box on a prescription blank to indicate to a pharmacist that a drug be dispensed in non-complying or non-child-resistant packaging.
    a. True
    b. False

29. Regarding insulin, which of the following is/are true?
    a. The only difference between the strength of U-100 insulin and U-500 insulin is the volume of liquid per milliliter which contains the insulin.
    b. All insulin container labels must include the words "Shake Well."
    c. U-100 insulin requires a physician's prescription because it is an injectable substance.
    d. Answers a and b are true.
    e. Answers b and c are true.

Matching: Determine the proper expiration dating for Questions 30 to 34.
    Use today's date.
    Use the following answer key.
    You may use some answers for more than one question.
    a. 1 year
    b. 2 years
    c. 5 years
    d. 3 months
    e. 6 months

30. You are filling a prescription for Valium in a community pharmacy. The expiration date on the manufacturer's container is 05/02. What expiration date should be used?

31. A patient calls your pharmacy and tells you that he has a bottle of insulin that has been stored, unopened in the refrigerator for awhile. He wants to know if it is still good to use. You feel that the storage conditions were okay. The expiration date on the bottle is 04/01. You tell him it's fine because the expiration date for insulin is _____.

32. You work in a hospital pharmacy. The pharmacy buys lanoxin tablets in bottles of 5000 because it is cheaper. You need to repackage it into single-use, unit-dose blister or bubble packs. The expiration date on the manufacturer's bottle is 01/2002. What expiration date should be used?

33. A patient comes into your pharmacy and asks how long drugs that drug companies sell to pharmacies are good for. You tell the patient that as long as proper storage conditions are met and the bottles remain unopened, the drug companies usually give medications about _____.

34. A patient brings a prescription into your community pharmacy for an eye drop used to treat glaucoma. The manufacturer's expiration date on the dropper bottle is 07/01. What expiration date should you use on the prescription label?

35. A(n)_____ is filed in order to permit generic copies of off-patent brand-name drugs easier access to the market.
    a. NDA
    b. INDA
    c. ANDA
    d. SNDA
    e. DNDA

36. A(n) _____ is filed to permit pharmaceutical companies to change the indications or dosage form for a drug or make a change in its manufacturing process.
    a. NDA
    b. INDA
    c. ANDA
    d. SNDA
    e. DNDA

37. What of the following is/are true regarding NDC numbers?
    a. If a label on a manufacturer's container has an NDC number on it, one can assume that the product requires a prescription.
    b. Product labels on OTC drugs can have NDC numbers on them.
    c. FDA requires all manufacturers to place an NDC number on all product labels.
    d. Answers a and b are true.
    e. Answers b and c are true.

38. Your pharmacy receives a letter from a pharmaceutical manufacturer which states that it is conducting a recall of a certain product because of reports that the product is causing self-limiting, mild rashes due to a color additive in about 10% of patients who take it. The letter also states that the problem is not dangerous to patients who are currently using it, but should no longer be dispensed to other patients. How would you characterize this incident?
    a. Class I, consumer level
    b. Class II, wholesale level
    c. Class II, retail level
    d. Class III, retail level
    e. Class III, consumer level

39. If this does not appear on a written prescription for phenobarbital, the prescription should not be filled by the pharmacist.

    a. Federal legend
    b. Expiration dates
    c. DEA number
    d. Federal transfer label
    e. NDC number

40. Products whose labeling is incorrect but are not contaminated are considered to be _____ but not _____.
    a. Misdirected, inconsistent
    b. Misbranded, adulterated
    c. Adulterated, misbranded
    d. Misbranded, USP
    e. USP, misbranded

41. Which of the following DEA numbers is correct for Doctor Ana Quinones?
    a. AQ 3798610
    b. RQ 1221390
    c. AA 1221388
    d. BQ 8139630
    e. AA 1256734

part four

DEA forms

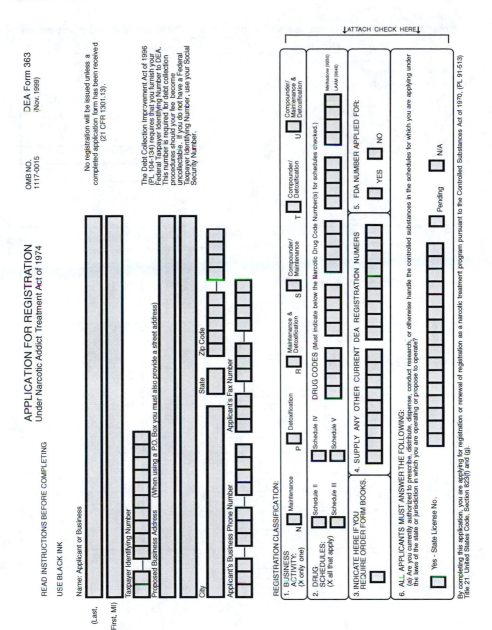

OMB Approval No. 1117 - 0007	U. S. Department of Justice / Drug Enforcement Administration **REGISTRANTS INVENTORY OF DRUGS SURRENDERED**	PACKAGE NO.

The following schedule is an inventory of controlled substances which is hereby surrendered to you for proper disposition.

FROM: *(Include Name, Street, City, State and ZIP Code in space provided below.)*

Signature of applicant or authorized agent

Registrant's DEA Number

Registrant's Telephone Number

NOTE: CERTIFIED MAIL (Return Receipt Requested) IS REQUIRED FOR SHIPMENTS OF DRUGS VIA U.S. POSTAL SERVICE. See instructions on reverse (page 2) of form.

NAME OF DRUG OR PREPARATION Registrants will fill in Columns 1,2,3, and 4 ONLY.	Number of Con-tainers	CONTENTS (Number of grams, tablets, ounces or other units per con-tainer)	Con-trolled Sub-stance Con-tent, (Each Unit)	FOR DEA USE ONLY		
				DISPOSITION	QUANTITY	
					GMS.	MGS.
1	*2*	*3*	*4*	*5*	*6*	*7*
1						
2						
3						
4						
5						
6						
7						
8						
9						
10						
11						
12						
13						
14						
15						
16						

FORM DEA-41 (9-01)   Previous edition dated **6-86** is usable.   *See instructions on reverse (page 2) of form.*

U.S. Department of Justice
Drug Enforcement Administration

**REPORT OF THEFT OR LOSS
OF CONTROLLED SUBSTANCES**

Federal Regulations require registrants to submit a detailed report of any theft or loss of Controlled Substances to the Drug Enforcement Administration.

Complete the front and back of this form in triplicate. Forward the original and duplicate copies to the nearest DEA Office. Retain the triplicate copy for your records. Some states may also require a copy of this report.

OMB APPROVAL
No. 1117-0001

1. Name and Address of Registrant (include ZIP Code)

ZIP CODE

2. Phone No. (Include Area Code)

3. DEA Registration Number

2 ltr. prefix   7 digit suffix

4. Date of Theft or Loss

5. Principal Business of Registrant (Check one)

1 ☐ Pharmacy   5 ☐ Distributor
2 ☐ Practitioner   6 ☐ Methadone Program
3 ☐ Manufacturer   7 ☐ Other (Specify)
4 ☐ Hospital/Clinic

6. County in which Registrant is located

7. Was Theft reported to Police?

☐ Yes   ☐ No

8. Name and Telephone Number of Police Department (Include Area Code)

9. Number of Thefts or Losses Registrant has experienced in the past 24 months

10. Type of Theft or Loss (Check one and complete items below as appropriate)

1 ☐ Night break-in   3 ☐ Employee pilferage   5 ☐ Other (Explain)
2 ☐ Armed robbery   4 ☐ Customer theft   6 ☐ Lost in transit (Complete Item 14)

11. If Armed Robbery, was anyone:

Killed? ☐ No   ☐ Yes (How many) _____
Injured? ☐ No ☐ Yes (How many) _____

12. Purchase value to registrant of Controlled Substances taken?

$

13. Were any pharmaceuticals or merchandise taken?

☐ No   ☐ Yes (Est. Value)

$

14. IF LOST IN TRANSIT, COMPLETE THE FOLLOWING:

A. Name of Common Carrier

B. Name of Consignee

C. Consignee's DEA Registration Number

D. Was the carton received by the customer?

☐ Yes   ☐ No

E. If received, did it appear to be tampered with?

☐ Yes   ☐ No

F. Have you experienced losses in transit from this same carrier in the past?

☐ No   ☐ Yes (How Many) _____

15. What identifying marks, symbols, or price codes were on the labels of these containers that would assist in identifying the products?

16. If Official Controlled Substance Order Forms (DEA-222) were stolen, give numbers.

17. What security measures have been taken to prevent future thefts or losses?

PRIVACY ACT INFORMATION

AUTHORITY: Section 301 of the Controlled Substances Act of 1970 (PL 91-513).
PURPOSE: Report theft or loss of Controlled Substances.
ROUTINE USES: The Controlled Substances Act authorizes the production of special reports required for statistical and analytical purposes. Disclosures of information from this system are made to the following categories of users for the purposes stated:

A. Other Federal law enforcement and regulatory agencies for law enforcement and regulatory purposes.
B. State and local law enforcement and regulatory agencies for law enforcement and regulatory purposes.

EFFECT: Failure to report theft or loss of controlled substances may result in penalties under Section 402 and 403 of the Controlled Substances Act.

Under the Paperwork Reduction Act, a person is not required to respond to a collection of information unless it displays a currently valid OMB control number.
Public reporting burden for this collection of information is estimated to average 30 minutes per response, including the time for reviewing instructions, searching existing data sources, gathering and maintaining the data needed, and completing and reviewing the collection of information. Send comments regarding this burden estimate or any other aspect of this collection of information, including suggestions for reducing this burden, to the Records Management Section, Drug Enforcement Administration, Washington, D.C. 20537; and to the Office of Information and Regulatory Affairs, Office of Management and Budget, Washington, D.C. 20503.

DEA Form - 106
(Dec. 1985)

Previous edition dated 03/83 Is OBSOLETE

CONTINUE ON REVERSE

DEA FORM-222
U.S. OFFICIAL ORDER FORM - SCHEDULES I & II

See Reverse of PURCHASER'S Copy of Instructions	No order form may be issued for Schedule I and II substances unless a completed application form has been received. (21 CFR 1305 04).		**OMB APROVAL No. 1117-0010**
TO: *(Name of Supplier)*	STREET ADDRESS		
CITY and STATE	DATE	**TO BE FILLED IN BY SUPPLIER**	
		SUPPLIERS DEA REGISTRATION No.	

L I N E No.	TO BE FILLED IN BY PURCHASER					
	No. of Packages	Size of Package	Name of Item	National Drug Code	Packages Shipped	Date Shipped
1						
2						
3						
4						
5						
6						
7						
8						
9						
10						

◄ **LAST LINE COMPLETED** *(MUST BE 10 OR LESS)*   SIGNATURE OF PURCHASER OR ATTORNEY OR AGENT

Date Issued	DEA Registration No.	Name and Address of Registrant
Schedules		
Registered as a	No. of this Order Form	

DEA Form-222
(Oct. 1992)

U.S. OFFICIAL ORDER FORMS - SCHEDULES I & II
DRUG ENFORCEMENT ADMINISTRATION
SUPPLIER'S Copy 1

Index

UNIVERSITY OF RHODE ISLAND

3 1222 01013 132 7

REF KF 2915 .P4 P57 2003
Pisano, Douglas J.
Essentials of pharmacy law

NO LONGER THE PROPERTY
OF THE
UNIVERSITY OF RI LIBRARY